Behavioral Genetics

Behavioral Genetics
The Clash of Culture and Biology

Edited by

Ronald A. Carson

Harris L. Kempner Distinguished Professor
in the Humanities in Medicine
Director, Institute for the Medical Humanities
University of Texas Medical Branch at Galveston
Galveston, Texas

and Mark A. Rothstein

Hugh Roy and Lillie Cranz Cullen
Distinguished Professor of Law
Director, Health Law and Policy Institute
University of Houston
Houston, Texas

The Johns Hopkins University Press
Baltimore and London

© 1999 The Johns Hopkins University Press
All rights reserved. Published 1999
Printed in the United States of America on acid-free paper
9 8 7 6 5 4 3 2 1

The Johns Hopkins University Press
2715 North Charles Street
Baltimore, Maryland 21218-4363
www.press.jhu.edu

Library of Congress Cataloging-in-Publication Data

Behavioral genetics : the clash of culture and biology / edited by
    Ronald A. Carson and Mark A. Rothstein.
        p.   cm.
    Includes bibliographical references and index.
    ISBN 0-8018-6069-5 (alk. paper)
    1. Behavior genetics.   I. Carson, Ronald A., 1940–
    II. Rothstein, Mark A.
    QH457.B44   1999
    616.89′042—dc21   98-43307
                                                             CIP

A catalog record for this book is available from the British Library.

Contents

Foreword

As a medically trained neuroscientist, my lifelong approach to diseases of the brain and behavior has been to search deeper and deeper into the causal mechanisms and points of biological vulnerability. Medical scientists frequently employ vertical thinking, which in terms of the brain and its disorders is a much richer expression than the "reductionist" appellation frequently used to cast aspersions of simple-mindedness onto biologists who rarely bother with psychosocial causes of illness. By thinking vertically, I am not satisfied just with finding genes that may mark vulnerability or resistance to a disease. Rather, I want to understand how the products of that gene, expressed selectively or ubiquitously, or somewhere in between, can influence neurons or glia; disregulate circuit formation or function; influence integrated functional systems; and change the way an individual interacts with, perceives, or anticipates the environment. Studies in which I have been a participant for more than fifteen years continue to strengthen the view that the brain relies on more genes to carry out its functions than any other organ in the body, and that more than half of the mammalian genome is of use to the brain. The Human Genome Project has already identified more than 40,000 bits of brain genes and I am thrilled at the information we will have on neuronal phenotypes and their functional variations once those initial discoveries have been characterized as to sites and times of expression.

In one of my longest-running fields of endeavor, namely, vulnerability to alcoholism, I have been impressed with the way family histories support the tendency for vulnerability to alcoholism to run in families, often with devastating influence, in a male-to-male transmission pattern. Being predisposed to accept the validity of that human pattern, I am further predisposed to accept the results of studies on rats bred to express greater and greater desire to drink alcohol and to show by their behavior that they will work to gain access to the alcohol. The data derived from the studies of these alcohol-preferring rodents also show comparable responses to drugs that help reduce alcohol ingestion and reduce recidivism in humans. Invasive studies of the alcoholic rats have revealed certain consistent alterations in brain neurochemistry and cellular function. However, there is still much to be learned before scientists will have a list of discrete gene expressions that will allow them to compare the alcohol-preferring animals and the alcohol-ignoring animals, let alone understand which combinations of changes may be the cause of the apparent simulation of the human alcoholic's condition.

Does this indicate that psychosocial factors and social culture have no bearing on the quest for understanding? No, not at all. When alcohol-preferring rats are placed in an environment in which they previously worked to obtain their alcoholic beverage, they begin to show the same neurochemical changes they showed when they were actively working to obtain alcohol. If these animals are never given a chance to drink, they clearly have no problems maintaining their simple existence and reproducing in laboratory settings.

Do I think there is only one gene "responsible" for alcoholism, or any other complex behavioral disease of emotion, cognition, or social interaction? Certainly not. I simply do not yet have a glimmer of the ways in which specific gene abnormalities of the sorts that are consistently observed in Huntington disease and that are occasionally observed in Alzheimer and Parkinson diseases can lead to the late-life devastations that characterize these untreatable pathologies. Those pathways need to be determined before we can have any prospects for understanding the still more variable biological bases by which some families show greatly increased incidences of other psychopathologies, and in which the consistent nonreproducibility of specific gene associations across such families suggests that there may be numerous routes to increased biological vulnerability.

Clearly, at present we have an incomplete genetic inventory of the brain and hence of the consequences for brain assembly, homeostatic adaptation, ability and desire to learn, and whatever goes into resilience to internal and external stressors. Nevertheless, this ignorance is slowly being reduced, and the only clash I see is with those who would take the view that the rich biology of the brain is irrelevant to the causes of mental diseases, or to their cure or ultimate prevention. In my view, this strategy does not have the remotest chance of success. Yet as scholars, we are required to keep an open mind, to be willing to hear and assess a variety of data as well as concepts and hypotheses, and then, if sufficiently challenged, to find ways to test those hypotheses. As this book amply demonstrates, there are many contrasting views and much data to be gathered if contrasting views of the causes of behavioral disorders are to be unified.

Floyd E. Bloom, M.D.
Department of Neuropharmacology
The Scripps Research Institute
La Jolla, California

Preface and Acknowledgments

Modern science is a product of Western culture. Its practitioners and laypersons alike take for granted culture-specific conceptions of self and society, freedom, responsibility, and human flourishing. Current developments in genetics are prompting a reevaluation of those ideas and a reconsideration of what constitutes responsible use of new knowledge.

The Human Genome Project is proceeding on schedule, with experts predicting that the entire genome sequence will be completed no later than 2005. Much of the scientific attention has already shifted away from single-gene disorders, such as cystic fibrosis, to complex disorders, such as various cancers. Lurking only slightly away from the glare of attention, however, like an uninvited guest sitting in a corner, are thorny issues surrounding behavioral genetics.

Genetic diseases have understandably garnered most of the attention so far. The promise that pernicious and intractable human diseases could be identified in advance and treated, or even prevented, has supplied the moral power to drive the engine of the Human Genome Project. However, important ethical, legal, and social issues are being raised in determining how our health care system will respond to new genetic discoveries. The issues include access to technology, genetic counseling, reproductive freedom, informed consent, and the role of genetics in public health. The use of genetic information for nonmedical purposes, such as insurance, employment, domestic relations, and forensics, has spurred a reexamination of notions of privacy and confidentiality.

Claims of genetic factors in behavior have been slower to develop. Indeed, genetic research on mental illness, for example, often has been characterized by false premises, unreplicated claims, and retracted papers. There are many reasons for this, including the difficulty of establishing diagnostic criteria, complex modes of inheritance, multiple gene interactions, difficulty in measuring end points, problems of methodology, and the uncertain effects of environment. These research problems are intensified for nonpathological behavioral factors. Nevertheless, assertions of a genetic link to thrill seeking, aggression, nurturing, aging, the development of language and social skills in women, "handedness," and food preferences all have been announced recently. Sexual orientation, alcoholism and other addictive behavior, and intelligence have surfaced to varying degrees as well. Our individual and collective responses to these emerging scientific claims will go to the heart of future societal and human relations.

One can take up the challenges of behavioral genetics by analyzing the issues from two different but related perspectives. If a scientific claim involving behavioral genetics is flawed, the initial solution consists of exposing errors in the scientific theory or method underlying the claim. Scientific refutation, however, is not the end of the matter. Even discredited scientific claims, once disseminated by the media, sometimes take on a life of their own.

For scientifically valid claims about behavioral genetics, which are likely to increase significantly in the years ahead, the issues are more complex. The nature of the claims and the uses to be made of the scientific connection are mere starting points. Where the science is good, we must determine what responses are socially appropriate and ethically defensible.

Either way, dispassionate analysis is difficult in today's political and intellectual climate. A controversial meeting in Maryland a few years ago on the genetic origins of criminal behavior touched off a storm of public protests. *The Bell Curve's* assertion of a racial variation in the genetic component of intelligence and the authors' proposed political response made for one of the most controversial books of the past decade (Herrnstein and Murray 1994).

As the editor of *Nature* noted several years ago, "Part of the trouble is that the excitement of the chase of molecular cause leaves little time for reflection. And there are grants for producing data, but hardly any for standing back in contemplation" (Maddox 1988). The collaborative project from which this book has emerged was an exercise in "standing back in contemplation." The idea for this volume arose out of an interdisciplinary dialogue about culture and biology. A grant from the John D. and Catherine T. MacArthur Foundation to the University of Texas Medical Branch's Institute for the Medical Humanities enabled a group of scholars in the biological, behavioral, and social sciences, the humanities, and law to bring interdisciplinary perspectives to bear on pressing questions arising at the intersection of culture and biology.

The chapters in this book suggest the need for a more sweeping series of dialogues on scientific and social perspectives, both among disciplines and among the public. The interdisciplinary dialogues should involve discussions of research goals, hypotheses, methodologies, conclusions, and implications. The public dialogues should focus on critical analysis of scientific claims, putting behavioral genetic developments in context, and using behavioral genetics responsibly and sensitively in formulating public policy.

The contributors to this volume are all experts in their respective fields, and their views would all be considered within the mainstream of their disciplines. Yet the variation among disciplines is striking in several ways: in their confidence in the validity of scientific claims of present and future association of genetics and behavior, in the level of concern about the possible misuse of genetic information, and in their assessment of the societal challenges in responding to proven associations between genetics and behavior.

Allan Tobin likens genetic determinism to earlier notions of predestination, noting that genetic boosterism conveniently accounts for worldly success and failure as unfortunate but not unjust because they are foreordained. He avers that only those for whom genetic information is an abstraction are likely to find genetic determinism appealing. Those at risk for disease are less sanguine. Tobin calls for research to deepen our understanding of gene-environment interactions in complex behaviors.

David Rowe and Kristen Jacobson observe that there is such widespread acceptance of the field of behavioral genetics by psychologists and psychiatrists that it is considered "mainstream" research. Nevertheless, other social scientists, such as cultural anthropologists and sociologists, largely ignore the substantial scientific evidence that has been developed. Using twin and adoption studies, kinship studies, and other traditional methods of inquiry, Rowe and Jacobson review current research directions in psychological and psychiatric uses of genetic findings for understanding behavioral development. Increased methodological rigor and new insights from molecular biology promise to increase the wider acceptance of behavioral genetics.

In their discussion of the molecular genetic basis of behavioral traits, Stephanie Sherman and Irwin Waldman describe current methods for finding genes for complex traits. They use schizophrenia, dyslexia, and anxiety as examples of successful investigations of the molecular basis of human behavior. The authors point to major advances in isolating the biological from the environmental components of complex behavioral traits.

Kenneth Schaffner enriches our appreciation for the complexity of behavioral genetics by replacing simple genetic reductionist models with interpretations of recent molecular advances. He points out that much of the interest in psychiatric genetics is predicated on the (false) hope that it may be possible to identify genes that contribute to serious mental disorders and that the information thus generated may then be used to treat those disorders. Schaffner counsels against the seductiveness of such a single-gene approach and argues instead for an intermingled set of approaches to mental disorders.

According to Mark Rothstein's analysis, law has tended to contribute to the legitimization of genetic determinism by failing to respond critically to misguided scientific and societal forces. Not only has the legislative process been susceptible to pressure to codify the prevailing social and cultural milieu, but also historically the courts have offered little resistance. As for new issues in behavioral genetics, Rothstein expresses concern about whether the combination of the adversary system, inexpert judges, lay juries, the lack of medical privacy, and other factors will contribute to the misuse of behavioral genetics in various legal settings.

Continuing the line of reasoning initiated by Rothstein, Lori Andrews explores the use of behavioral genetics by the criminal justice system. She probes the reasons for increased interest in evidence of genetic propensities to commit antisocial acts and describes the justifications for assigning legal responsibility and meting out punishment for such acts. Andrews' analysis raises the specter of how the legal system might respond to genetic predictions in the absence of a crime. If genetic propensities to criminal behavior are discoverable in retrospect, what is to prevent prospective intervention to identify potential future law breakers, place them under surveillance or in preventive detention, and perhaps provide them with social or medical treatment?

Dorothy Nelkin takes up a theme briefly broached in this volume by Allan Tobin, namely, the popular appeal of genetic explanations in mass culture (Nelkin and Lindee 1995). She inquires into the public policy implications of construing social problems in terms of an ostensibly national predisposition of individuals to behave in certain ways. Nelkin shows how genetic explanations of human behavior can be appropriated by various social, political, and economic ideologies. In the context of dismantling the welfare state, she argues, "scientific concepts concerning the heritability of behavior have been translated into a rhetoric of responsibility and blame which purports to account for such phenomena as antisocial behavior, educational failure, and social inequities." In Nelkin's view, the popularity of behavioral genetics is in large measure attributable to the character of the current political climate.

For his exploration of the social construction of genetic information, Troy Duster focuses on concrete situations of disclosure. By means of a cross-cultural analysis, he demonstrates the indelibly local and ethnic character of social meaning. Even "individual choice" is socially situated and culture specific, which is why voluntarism is a fundamentally contested concept and coercion an ever-present danger. Echoing a view expressed in this volume by Lori Andrews and Mark Rothstein, Duster cautions against what he calls "creeping geneticism," whereby molecular genetic knowledge intended for the prevention of disease and the improvement of health is enlisted in the service of the criminal justice system and used in hiring and insurance decisions.

Ronald Carson takes up the question of how to maintain one's moral bearings in a genetic age in which the self is caught in a tension between fate and mastery. He proposes a broad-gauged, inclusive dialogue to discern what constitutes acceptable risk and responsible action under conditions of uncertainty and irreversibility.

In addition to the authors represented in this volume, the editors wish to acknowledge other valuable contributors to the Culture and Biology project: Michele A. Carter, P. Michael Conneally, Joseph T. Boyle, John Douard, Helen Donis-Keller, S. Van McCrary, Ellen S. More, Rebecca D. Pentz, Martin S. Pernick, Robert M. Rose, Lee S. Rowen, Gunter S. Stent, T. Howard Stone, William D. Willis Jr., and William J. Winslade.

Our sincere thanks to Diane Pfeil for preparing the manuscript and managing the editorial process; to Faith Lagay and Sara Clausen for expert editorial assistance; to Sharon Goodwin for managing the project; and to Lori Helton for seeing it through to successful completion.

Finally, we express our gratitude to the John D. and Catherine T. MacArthur Foundation and especially to the foundation's director of Mental Health Policy and Research Program on Human and Community Development, Robert M. Rose, M.D., who made the project and this publication possible.

References

Herrnstein, R. J., and C. Murray. 1994. *The Bell Curve: Intelligence and Class Structure in American Life.* New York: Free Press.

Maddox, J. 1988. Finding wood among the trees. *Nature* 333:11.

Nelkin, D., and M. S. Lindee. 1995. *The DNA Mystique: The Gene as a Cultural Icon.* New York: Freeman.

Contributors

Lori B. Andrews, J.D., Professor of Law, Chicago-Kent College of Law, and Director, Institute for Science, Law, and Technology, Illinois Institute of Technology, Chicago, Illinois

Troy Duster, Ph.D., Director, Institute for the Study of Social Change, University of California at Berkeley, Berkeley, California

Kristen C. Jacobson, M.S., doctoral candidate, Department of Human Development and Family Studies, Pennsylvania State University, University Park, Pennsylvania

Dorothy Nelkin, University Professor of the Social Sciences, Department of Sociology and School of Law, New York University, New York

David C. Rowe, Ph.D., Professor of Family Studies, University of Arizona, Tucson, Arizona

Kenneth F. Schaffner, M.D., Ph.D., University Professor of Medical Humanities, George Washington University, Washington, D.C.

Stephanie L. Sherman, Ph.D., Professor, Department of Genetics, Emory University School of Medicine, Atlanta, Georgia

Allan J. Tobin, Ph.D., Eleanor Leslie Chair in Neuroscience and Neurology, and Director, Brain Research Institute, University of California at Los Angeles, Los Angeles, California

Irwin Douglas Waldman, Ph.D., Associate Professor, Department of Psychology, Emory University, Atlanta, Georgia

Behavioral Genetics

1 Amazing Grace

Sources of Phenotypic Variation in Genetic Boosterism

Allan J. Tobin, Ph.D.

Enthusiasm for Genetics Has Decreased among People at Risk for Disease

In July 1983, I helped organize a Hereditary Disease Foundation workshop at the University of Rochester on the clinical implications of genetic testing. The fifteen workshop participants included geneticists, neurologists, and genetic counselors. The discussions were to be speculative—what would be the implications for clinical practice if new DNA-based methods made it possible to predict who would get a late-onset genetic disease, such as Huntington disease? The Hereditary Disease Foundation had already been pushing the application of molecular genetics to Huntington disease, but the Rochester workshop was our first attempt to explore how genetics might change the clinical practice of neurology.

No one thought the discussion would be tied to the immediate reality of disease prediction. However, two weeks before the workshop, James Gusella discovered that a DNA polymorphism was closely linked to the disease locus in two families with Huntington disease, one from the U.S. Midwest and one from the shores of Venezuela's Lake Maracaibo. The odds against Gusella's finding being explainable merely by chance were 100,000,000 to 1 (Gusella et al. 1983).

As a result of Gusella's still-unpublished discovery, we all believed that finding the linkage marker meant that finding the gene itself was only a few steps away, and we thought and hoped that a cure could not be far behind. It did not occur to us that it would take a ten-year effort and some fifty researchers to find the gene itself (Huntington's Disease Collaborative Research Group 1993). Nor did we worry that once the gene was found, we would not know what it did or how to intervene in its action. In July 1983, most of our talk focused on the freedom that would come to a person at risk for Huntington disease. Finally he or she would be able to plan—to have children, to start a business, to become an astronaut.

As the discussion continued, however, I became depressed. I realized that predictions for a dominant disease would bring equal measures of good and bad news for the people I knew to be at risk. I thought of the questions I used to ask at-risk family members who came to Hereditary Disease Foundation workshops: "Would you personally want to know if you were carrying the disease-causing gene? Would you take the test, once it was developed?" Everyone said, "Yes, certainly. I would want to know, either way." Yet only a small fraction (about 5% in several surveys) of at-risk individuals who have been offered a chance to take the test have actually chosen to take it (Kessler et al. 1987; Quaid and Morris 1993).

As was the case for Huntington disease, the bumpy search for genes underlying schizophrenia and bipolar disease has evoked varying psychological responses from people on the front line—those whose families are directly affected. Until 1979, at the beginning of the excitement about the power of molecular genetics for predicting diseases of the brain, organizations that represented families of the mentally ill were relatively small. This lack of cohesiveness was not surprising in view of widespread stigmatization: a commonly argued causal factor for schizophrenia was bad parenting, as expressed in the concept of the schizophrenogenic mother. The idea that genes—not parenting practices—cause schizophrenia was enthusiastically welcomed, and the National Alliance for the Mentally Ill now has 140,000 members. A genetic view of etiology provided more than hope for advances in research: it offered both private and public exculpation for being ill. Still, I doubt that if schizophrenia "genes" are ever found the relatives of people with schizophrenia will line up to be tested.

Why has the enthusiasm for genetics decreased among people at risk for Huntington disease and increased among the families of people with schizophrenia? Why do biologists differ so strikingly in their thoughts about the genetic determinants of behavior? Why are neuroscientists and traditional developmental biologists generally more skeptical about genetic determinism than molecular geneticists? Why should anyone brought up on Western ideas of free will embrace any kind of deterministic thinking? And why did *The Bell Curve*, a long and technical book, make it to the *New York Times* bestseller list (Herrnstein and Murray 1994; Fraser 1995)?

Clearly, a gap exists between the perceptions of people for whom the significance of genetic information is most immediate (those at risk for a familial disease) and those for whom genetic information is abstract. Surveys of at-risk individuals and physicians underscore this difference: physicians are less convinced of the importance of pretest and post-test counseling than are at-risk people themselves (Wertz and Fletcher 1989; Thomassen et al. 1993). For physicians, genetic tests are like any other diagnostic tool, but for people at risk, they lead literally to life-and-death decisions. In one case, for example, a genetic diagnosis for Huntington disease, delivered over the telephone, was the immediate stimulus for suicide.

I have been trying to understand the sources of varying attitudes toward genetics in the context of what is known about the interactions of genes, environment, and experience. I am particularly concerned about how the public perceives the role of genetics in intelligence, violence, homosexuality, and other complex behaviors (Fraser 1995). How have the paradigms of molecular biologists and the public's hunger for simple deterministic answers played into one another? I suggest that psychological, intellectual, political, and even religious differences have shaped the scientific and public debates over the genetics of behavior.

Why Is Genetic Enthusiasm High among Experimental Biologists?

Phenotype is the set of properties that we can observe when we examine a person or organism. Phenotype includes appearance and chemistry—size and shape, color and smell. The phenotypic traits that compelled Gregor Mendel's attention included the size of his pea plants and the colors of their flowers; those noticed by Thomas Hunt Morgan included the eye color and wing venations of *Drosophila;* those most noticed in the human population range from size and skin color to specific illnesses such as Huntington disease.

Every population contains enormous phenotypic variation. The first recorded application of a strategy to reduce this genetic variation is in the book of Genesis, which describes the patriarch Jacob breeding his spotted goats separately from his father-in-law's unspotted stock (Genesis 30: 32–43). However, long before the time of Jacob, pastoral and agricultural peoples must have recognized the need to select among genetically variant stocks—a recognition that continued and grew through the centuries. Science, which is ultimately concerned with the reproducibility of results, always seeks ways to eliminate variation in any study. Good experimental design requires that all the subjects of a study be exposed to the same environmental conditions, except for the limited number of experimental variables. Researchers in molecular and cell biology are especially careful to use highly inbred lines of animals and plants to minimize genetic variation.

Since the discovery of the nature of genes, biologists have had more concrete goals. We want to find *the* gene responsible for a particular phenotypic character. My own laboratory has contributed to this effort and identified several genes involved in the synthesis and action of the major inhibitory neurotransmitter, γ-aminobutyric acid (GABA) (Olsen and Tobin 1990; Erlander et al. 1991; Medina-Kauwe et al. 1994).

The genes that we sought had already been defined biochemically and pharmacologically, so our discoveries did not solve any mysteries about the relationship between genes and phenotypic traits. The reason for looking at GABA-related genes came from my previous interest in neurogenetic disorders, especially Huntington disease, in which GABA-producing cells are the first to die (Albin et al. 1989). After showing that none of the genes we found were altered in Huntington disease, we spent several years unsuccessfully looking for a neurological disease associated with GABA gene defects (Kaufman et al. 1990). We know that GABA is involved in the regulation of movements and seizures, but no diseases have been discovered.

Molecular geneticists have implicitly assumed that there is a canonical sequence for each gene (at least with respect to its ability to encode a specific protein) and that variations from that sequence are likely to be detrimental. Of course, every geneticist is aware of the existence of genetic variations, but most variations that persist in the population are phenotypically silent; in some cases they do not even change the sequence of amino acids in a protein. Geneticists are careful to talk nonjudgmentally about sequence variations from the "wild type," which has been defined in statistical, not normative, terms. However, at some level, most researchers have never really believed that variations are as good as the genes that we have sequenced ourselves, where wild-type sequences have the aura of platonic ideals.

As geneticists continue to discover disease-causing genes, they reinforce the notion that allelic variation means disease or at least dysfunction. The disease-causing genes that were found first encoded mutant hemoglobins, which cause sickle cell disease; phenylalanine hydroxylase (whose absence underlies phenylketonuria); and hexosaminidase (whose absence underlies Tay-Sachs disease). While everyone was aware that some sequence variations did not cause disease, the push was always to find the disease-causing mutations.

As these and other genes fell, geneticists expanded their quarry to genes whose biochemical identities were as yet unknown. With the emergence of positional cloning, molecular geneticists were able to find genes responsible for phenotypic traits that had been previously uncharacterized biochemically (Karch et al. 1985). Later, the discovery of DNA-based genetic markers allowed researchers to find genes responsible for human diseases—Duchenne muscular dystrophy, neurofibromatosis, cystic fibrosis, Huntington disease, and scores of others. Most of the diseases turned out to result from loss-of-function mutations in essential proteins, which is conceptually no different from the loss of function in phenylketonuria.

However, instead of talking about "disease-causing mutations," both molecular geneticists and the public who avidly followed their progress began to talk of "disease genes." Even the naming of positionally cloned genes reflected this shorthand: the protein that is defective in Duchenne muscular dystrophy was named "dystrophin" as if the disease established the protein's normal function. Similarly, we now have "huntingtin," "ataxin," and "cystic fibrosis transmembrane regulator." These successes and their attendant neologisms reinforced this reductionist views of genetics.

The ability to identify disease-causing genes by positional cloning has attracted the attention of both scientists and laypersons, for many good reasons. (1) Gene identification leads to diagnosis and identification of gene carriers. (2) Gene identification can distinguish people with distinct but phenotypically similar diseases, for example, in the ataxias. (3) Gene identification can lead directly to insights about pathogenesis, not only for the genetic forms of a disease, but also for sporadic cases, which geneticists may view as "phenocopies" of the genetic form. (4) Knowledge of pathogenesis can suggest new directions for prophylaxis and treatment. (5) Gene identification suggests possible direct interventions in the form of gene therapy (e.g., gene replacement in phenylketonuria or adenosine deaminase deficiency, or antisense strategies in genetic forms of cancer). These possibilities motivate the continuing search for other disease genes—a search that we must understand as just the first step, but which too often many people have seen as a hopeful end point.

Why Is Identification of a Gene Just the First Step in Understanding Phenotype?

A major task of genetics and developmental biology has been to define the relationships between genes and environment that give rise to phenotypes. Developmental biologists have sought to uncover the basis of these complex relationships, which may be called *epigenetic rules*.

Recently researchers have created their own loss-of-function mutations in mice, using techniques that "knock out" genes in the precursor cells of a mouse embryo (Capecchi 1989). The resulting embryo and mouse has a complete set of genes, except for the one targeted by the research. The results have been interesting but confusing, because gene after gene appears to be redundant—the majority of all knockout mice so far have a phenotype indistinguishable or barely distinguishable from the wild type. Other knockouts are lethal in embryonic development, and the particular pattern of embryonic death is often informative. So far, relatively few knockouts have produced clearly defined adult phenotypes, and many of those have been completely unforeseen, such as a mouse with angora fur, which resulted from the knock out of a growth factor (Hebert et al. 1994).

This murky picture is not a surprise to traditional developmental biologists, who have known all along about the uncertain and complex relationships between phenotype and genotype. What are some of the general epigenetic rules that have emerged from these studies?

1. Large numbers of genes interact to contribute to developmental programs.

Some mutations in some genes lead to major disruptions in development, but enormous genetic variation is tolerated without substantial effects on basic developmental programs (Waddington 1975). Indeed, widely divergent species in the same families, classes, and even phyla share the same developmental programs, as illustrated in the similar appearances of human, frog, and chick embryos.

2. Environmental factors are important.

A little acid in the water of the developing sea urchin will cause even the first step in its independent development (gastrulation) to go awry.

3. The influence of environment changes during development.

Early in development, cells removed from an amphibian embryo and transplanted into another cellular environment develop in accordance with their new, rather than their old, surround (Spemann 1938). Later (after gastrulation) this ability is lost, and transplanted cells stubbornly develop according to an already determined program. Developmental biologists have long known that timing is crucial, and that critical periods exist for the determination of cell fate.

Neuroscientists are also particularly aware of critical periods in development, for example, in the acquisition of language. Neuroscientists note that experience—which we consider an aspect of the environment—somehow writes on the brain, sometimes in indelible ink. We speak about the brain's *plasticity*, borrowing the word "plastic" from materials engineers. When an *elastic* material is deformed by some force, once the force has been released, it returns to its previous state. In contrast, a *plastic* material is permanently altered. In just this way, the brain is permanently altered by its experiences, during both embryonic and childhood development, and in adult life.

4. Even adults retain developmental flexibility.

Although the fates of many cells become fixed in early development, both cellular development and neural connections remain highly flexible. In gut, skin, blood, and even brain, adults harbor stem cells that are capable of reprogramming (Reynolds and Weiss 1992). The brain, of course, maintains its ability to learn, even in the face of hard-wired networks that influence our sensations, our actions, and even some of our thoughts.

5. Epigenetic rules are confounded by other factors.

Among the mind-bending concepts of chaos theory is the "butterfly wing effect," the idea that the fluttering of a butterfly's wings in Peking can affect storm systems in New York a month later (Gleick 1988). To this can be added the theories propounded by Frank Sulloway in *Born to Rebel* (Sulloway 1996). Sulloway contends that natural selection has favored allelic variants that promote sibling rivalry. He argues that birth order (rather than genes) significantly determines a person's pattern of thought, especially his or her willingness to embrace progressive or regressive revolutions.

Phenotype depends on both genes and environment, but (except for identical twins) every individual in an outbred population differs not only in the interaction among individual genes but also in the interactions between genes and environment. Even the particular ability to respond to environmental or experiential cues is part of the phenotype. That responsiveness, in turn, depends on genes, physical environment, and culture. Culture is important in nonhuman as well as human populations. The success of a famous macaque group in obtaining nourishment from its human protectors, for example, was forever changed when a young female discovered that she could separate rice from sand by flotation (Heyes and Galef 1996).

Many human diseases do not depend in any simple way on a single gene. Studies of twins have suggested that schizophrenia, for example, has a strong genetic component, but more than 50 percent of monozygotic twins are discordant for schizophrenia. A recent study suggests that monozygotic twins that do not share the same circulation are still more discordant, suggesting that the shared fetal environment (or shared fetal viral susceptibility) may be more important than genetics (Davis and Phelps 1995).

How Do Political and Religious Concerns Influence Attitudes toward Genetic Determinism?

We have seen the appeal of genetic determinism for molecular geneticists and the public. Why might social scientists and political pundits also embrace genetic determinism?

Genetics and molecular genetics pervade the Zeitgeist, but genetic boosterism (the unfettered enthusiasm for purely genetic explanations of medical, social, and even economic differences) is highly variable within the population. Anecdotal evidence suggests that it may run in families. This familial pattern is not altogether surprising: we know, for example, that religion and political party are among the most familial of all phenotypic traits (Lewontin 1982). As W. S. Gilbert put it, "Every boy and girl alive is either a little liberal or a little conservative."

Almost a century ago, Max Weber attributed the worldly success of Calvinist Protestants to the attempts by individual Calvinists to prove that they were foreordained recipients of divine grace (Weber 1991). Because humans had no way of knowing to whom God had extended the grace of salvation, Calvinists were plagued with unbearable insecurity, especially in the face of, to them, a literal hellfire. Weber argued that Calvinists desperately needed to find some way of making the divine will known to themselves. They found the answer in their own worldly success. The practical result was, in Weber's view, the most rapid possible accumulation of capital, making German Protestants far more successful than their Catholic compatriots. Calvinism, according to Weber, provided a way of escaping the guilt feelings that would otherwise come with success, since their success was deemed a sign of God's everlasting grace.

For many people—mostly those who do *not* spend their professional lives thinking about genes and environment—the appeal of genetic determinism appears similar to that of Calvinist grace: predestination (of whatever sort) means that no one is responsible for inequalities in society, for the success of some and the failures of others. Many secular contemporaries appear to be engaged in a similar enterprise to prove that they have been the foreordained recipients of good genes. We may reasonably wonder why so many academics argue so intensely about the excellence of their own genes.

Sadly, few experimental studies address issues that might actually contribute to the understanding of gene-environment interactions. The natural locus for this study should be in the brain itself. However, most of the ongoing work on neural plasticity and development focuses on simpler phenomena. Developmental biologists, especially developmental neurobiologists, should begin to look at genetic-environmental interactions in more complex behaviors. The proliferation of genetically variant inbred lines and of new methods for studying complex behaviors should make such research possible.

My own view is that for everlasting grace we should look not to our genes but to our own natural talents. However we acquired them—by genes, experience, or will—they are all we have. Some five hundred years ago, Pico della Mirandola summarized the powers and limitations of humans by putting the following words into the mouth of God, speaking to Adam just after Creation (Pico della Mirandola 1985): "We have made thee neither of heaven nor of earth, neither mortal nor immortal, so that with freedom of choice and with honor, as though the maker and molder of thyself, thou mayest fashion thyself in whatever shape thou shalt prefer."

References

Albin, R. L., A. B. Young, and J. B. Penney. 1989. The functional anatomy of basal ganglia disorders. *Trends Neurosci.* 12: 366–375.

Capecchi, M. R. 1989. Altering the genome by homologous recombination. *Science* 244: 1288–1292.

Davis, J. O., and J. A. Phelps. 1995. Twins with schizophrenia: genes or germs? *Schizophr. Bull.* 21: 13–18.

Erlander, M. G., N. J. K. Tillakaratne, S. Feldblum, et al. 1991. Two genes encode distinct glutamate decarboxylases. *Neuron* 7: 91–100.

Fraser, S., ed. 1995. *The Bell Curve Wars: Race, Intelligence, and the Future of America.* New York: Basic Books.

Gleick, J. 1988. *Chaos: Making a New Science.* New York: Penguin.

Gould, S. J. 1977. *Ontogeny and Phylogeny.* Cambridge, Mass.: Belknap Press of Harvard University Press.

Gusella, J. F., N. S. Wexler, P. M. Conneally, et al. 1983. A polymorphic DNA marker genetically linked to Huntington's disease. *Nature* 306: 234–238.

Hebert, J. M., T. Rosenquist, J. Gotz, and G. R. Martin. 1994. FGF5 as a regulator of the hair growth cycle: Evidence from targeted and spontaneous mutations. *Cell* 78: 1017–1025.

Herrnstein, R. J., and C. Murray. 1994. *The Bell Curve: Intelligence and Class Structure in American Life.* New York: Free Press.

Heyes, C. M., and B. G. Galef Jr., eds. 1996. *Social Learning in Animals: The Roots of Culture.* San Diego: Academic Press.

Huntington's Disease Collaborative Research Group. 1993. A novel gene containing a trinucleotide repeat that is expanded and unstable on Huntington's disease chromosomes. *Cell* 72: 971–983.

Karch, F., B. Weiffenbach, M. Peifer, et al. 1985. The abdominal region of the bithorax complex. *Cell* 43: 81–96.

Kaufman, D. L., V. Ramesh, A. I. McClatchey, et al. 1990. Detection of point mutations associated with genetic diseases by an exon scanning technique. *Genomics* 8: 656–663.

Kessler, S., T. Field, L. Worth, and H. Mosbarger. 1987. Attitudes of persons at risk for Huntington disease toward predictive testing. *Am. J. Med. Genet.* 26: 259–270.

Lewontin, R. C. 1982. *Human Diversity.* New York: Scientific American Library.

Medina-Kauwe, L. K., N. J. K. Tillakaratne, J. Y. Wu, and A. J. Tobin. 1994. A rat brain cDNA encodes enzymatically active GABA transaminase and provides a molecular probe for GABA-catabolizing cells. *J. Neurochem.* 62: 1267–1275.

Olsen, R. W., and A. J. Tobin. 1990. Molecular biology of GABA$_A$ receptors. *FASEB J.* 4: 1469–1480.

Pico della Mirandola, G. 1985. *On the Dignity of Man.* Charles Glenn Wallis, trans. New York: Macmillan.

Quaid, K. A., and M. Morris. 1993. Reluctance to undergo predictive testing: the case of Huntington disease. *Am. J. Med. Genet.* 45: 41–45.

Reynolds, B. A., and S. Weiss. 1992. Generation of neurons and astrocytes from isolated cells of the adult mammalian central nervous system. *Science* 255: 1707–1710.

Spemann, H. 1938. *Embryonic Development and Induction.* New Haven, Conn.: Yale University Press.

Sulloway, F. J. 1996. *Born to Rebel: Birth Order, Family Dynamics, and Creative Lives.* New York: Pantheon.

Thomassen, R., A. Tibben, M. F. Niermeijer, E. et al. 1993. Attitudes of Dutch general practitioners towards presymptomatic DNA-testing for Huntington disease. *Clin. Genet.* 43: 63–68.

Waddington, C. H. 1975. *The Evolution of an Evolutionist.* Edinburgh: Edinburgh University Press.

Weber, M. 1991. *The Protestant Ethic and the Spirit of Capitalism,* Talcott Parsons, trans.; Anthony Giddens, introduction. London: HarperCollins Academic.

Wertz, D. C., and J. C. Fletcher. 1989. An international survey of attitudes of medical geneticists toward mass screening and access to results. *Public Health Rep.* 104: 35–44.

2 In the Mainstream
Research in Behavioral Genetics

David C. Rowe, Ph.D., and
Kristen C. Jacobson, Ph.D.

Behavioral genetics is a field concerned with variation, with why one individual differs from another. One hypothesis holds that genetic differences among people are a source of their behavioral differences. The acceptance of this hypothesis differs across disciplines. In fields such as cultural anthropology and sociology, it is largely rejected or ignored. In other disciplines, such as psychiatry and psychology, the concept of genetic influence on behavior is entirely mainstream. Some branches of psychiatry are engaged in a veritable "gene hunt" for the genetic sources of psychiatric disorders their practitioners believe to be heritable. In psychology, behavioral genetics findings are published in the field's major journals and widely cited.

In her 1986 address to the Behavior Genetics Association, Sandra Scarr gave three cheers for behavioral genetics—one for juxtaposing "genetics" and "behavior," one for drawing attention to evolution, and one for persuading psychologists to take the genetics of behavior seriously. She foresaw that behavioral genetics was "in danger of being swallowed in a flood of acceptance" (Scarr 1987, 228). Although the acceptance of behavioral genetics is now so extensive that the field can celebrate its victories, it is also far from complete. Although it is always hazardous to venture a prediction, until more people become better informed about behavioral genetics, it is likely to continue as a distinct field instead of being, as anticipated by Scarr, swallowed up by other disciplines.

This chapter presents the advantages of using behavioral genetic designs to explain and predict behavior. First, we briefly consider the historical and scientific forces that led behavioral genetics to its current state of acceptance by many social scientists in most disciplines. Second, we discuss the estimation of variance components in behavioral genetics. Third, we review current research directions, focusing on those that employ traditional research designs (e.g., twin and adoption studies). (Chapter 3 in this volume covers current efforts to identify "genes for behavior" using molecular genetic techniques.) We close by considering one controversy in the field: the debate about shared environmental influences on behavior.

A Historical Look at the Acceptance of Behavioral Genetics

As we have mentioned, cultural anthropology and sociology reject or ignore concepts relating to the heritability of behavioral traits and downplay biological theory and data. At a recent meeting of the American Sociological Association, for example, none of the numerous sessions about gender, that is, male versus female differences in behavior, presented biological data or theory related to gender, such as hormonal influences on behavior or the evolutionary theory of ultimate causation. One cannot expect behavioral genetics to make inroads in these fields until biology has been given its due. With most graduate programs failing to provide exposure to the findings of behavioral genetics and training in its methods, it is understandable that progress toward the acceptance of behavioral genetics in these two disciplines has been slow. The hostility may well arise from a lack of understanding about the field.

In psychiatry and psychology, on the other hand, the growth in the acceptance of behavioral genetics has been enormous since the post–World War II period to the present. In her presidential address, Scarr cited political and economic changes as one cause for the greater acceptance of behavioral genetics. "Surely, the intellectual pendulum swings from the Watsonian view that a child can be made into anything the parents desire to a Gesellian view of individual development as internally guided. Today, expert opinion lies more with contemporary scientific and public opinions. The source of such shifts in opinion lies more with the political and economic tides than with science per se" (Scarr 1987, 228). Although Scarr emphasized forces external to behavioral genetics, we believe that forces *internal* to the field played an equal, if not greater, role in its acceptance by social science.

Behavioral genetics was founded by Francis Galton in the second half of the nineteenth century (Crow 1993). Galton made numerous contributions to science, including pressure bars in meteorology and fingerprinting in forensics. His major contributions to behavioral genetics include an appreciation of traits as continuous, the discovery of the concepts of correlation and regression (which form the basis of statistics), and the first use of family, twin, and adoption research designs. In his writings, however, Galton was unaware of

Mendelian genetics, which were rediscovered in 1900 (Galton died in 1911). It remained for Fisher (1918), who later held a chair in eugenics established by Galton at the University of London, to reconcile Mendelian genetics with quantitative (i.e., continuous trait) genetics. He did so by observing that although a single gene would yield only categorical traits (i.e., AA = yellow pea, Aa = yellow pea, aa = green pea), the action of multiple genes in concert would yield a smooth and continuous trait distribution (in which each gene has a relatively small effect on variation). Galton, too, inspired the social application of genetics in a movement called *eugenics* (meaning "well born") that sought to improve humanity through regulating human reproduction, much as artificial breeders improved nonhuman animal and plant species for human use.

In the period between 1930 and World War II, interest in genetic ideas in social science was already waning because of a dislike of eugenic policies and a belief that environmental change alone could solve social problems (see Degler 1991). Nazism, with its use of genetics as a justification for genocide, was the *coup de grâce* against genetic ideas in social science. However, as the Nazi abuse of genetics receded further into the past, an acceptance of behavioral genetics became more likely. As Scarr suggests, intellectual ideas sometimes swing much like a pendulum to extremes that require correction.

In addition to these external factors, we believe that ideas and findings within science have influenced the increased interest in behavioral genetics. Specifically, we believe that behavioral genetics' adoption findings on schizophrenia, its methodological critique of traditional family socialization studies, and its relation to the DNA revolution within biology all have contributed to its growing acceptance.

In the 1950s and early 1960s, the prevailing view of schizophrenia placed its etiology in ill-treatment by parents. In particular, mothers were blamed for fostering the illness in their children by their supposed emotional coldness and inconsistent discipline. This view fit well with the Freudian intellectual tradition that argued that small emotional slights early in a child's development could have devastating consequences at a later time. Watsonian and Skinnerian behaviorism also emphasized the family environment as the mold for child development. When a single theory is monolithic in a field, contrary findings can break paradigms (Kuhn 1962). It is just this role, we believe, that the first adoption studies of schizophrenia played in the 1960s, several years before the formation of the Behavior Genetics Association in 1970.

The earliest study was completed by Heston (1966). Although at that time most psychiatrists believed that inept mothers caused schizophrenia, Heston suspected, on the basis of his own cases, a genetic link in the transmission of schizophrenia. In particular, he noted a case in which a biological mother seemed perfectly competent, despite the psychological stresses of raising a schizophrenic child (see Plomin et al. 1997, 71). The child's mental illness therefore could not be attributed to poor parenting. Heston undertook a study that compared children born to schizophrenic mothers who were raised by adoptive parents with children born to nonschizophrenic mothers who were also raised by adoptive parents.

Of the 47 adopted-away children of schizophrenics, five were schizophrenic, and an additional three had some type of chronic mental illness. None of the 45 adopted-away children of normal mothers were schizophrenic. In addition, the 10 percent rate of schizophrenia seen in these at-risk children is similar to the overall rate of schizophrenia found in biological children raised by a schizophrenic mother, indicating that rearing by a schizophrenic adds little environmental effect. Although Heston's sample was small, later studies confirmed these general findings (Rowe 1994). His results, coming at a time of dominant environmentalism, stirred the Zeitgeist and gave impetus to the formation of the Behavior Genetics Association at the Institute for Behavior Genetics in Boulder, Colorado.

A second internal reason for the growth of respect for behavioral genetics within social science during the past three decades is its methodological integrity (Rowe 1994). The majority of studies of environmental effects examine associations between parental behavior and child outcomes in biological families. This design is flawed because it does not take genetic influence on behavior into account. Genes may affect parental behaviors (e.g., warmth toward a child, consistency of discipline) and copies of the same genes in children may affect their traits. With genetic effects operating in both generations, it may be spurious to associate parent-child behavioral traits with environmental influence. This major flaw in the traditional research design for family study renders social science research on "family environmental effects" ambiguous at best. As environmentally oriented researchers in psychiatry and psychology have accepted the limitations of the traditional family study design, they have come to embrace behavioral genetic research methods that separate genetic from environmental effects (e.g., Reiss 1995). In this way, behavioral genetics has moved out of the hands of researchers primarily interested in genes and their effects and into the hands of those interested in environmental effects.

A third force internal to science that has contributed to the increased acceptance of behavioral genetics is its tie to biology, especially molecular genetics. Since the structure of DNA was discovered by the American-English team of Watson and Crick in 1953, the pace of discovery of specific genes and their phenotypic effects has accelerated enormously. Behavioral genetics has benefited because genes, originally hypothetical constructs with no *directly* observable reality, have become real, quantifiable, and even manipulable. The scientific prestige of molecular biology has carried over to behavioral genetics as the possibility of finding genes connected to the variation of particular traits (called quantitative trait loci [QTL]) has become real.

The Estimation of Variance Components

Traditional behavioral genetics is about the estimation of variance components—that is, why people's behavior (as well as that of nonhuman animals) differs from one person to another. The cause of these differences may lie in genetic inheritance or in environmental influences. This is the long-standing nature-nurture distinction. More recently, the variance partitioning has become finer tuned, allowing investigators to distinguish between particular types of environmental effects and to identify the different mechanisms by which genes may be expressed and/or exert their effects on behavior.

Two types of environmental influence—shared and nonshared—are commonly distinguished in behavioral genetics. Shared environmental influences are those that (by definition) operate to make siblings similar to one another. Although simple on its surface, the concept of shared environment has some subtleties. Four conditions must be satisfied for an environmental effect to count as shared. First, near universals found within a culture may not be counted. For example, the English language is a near universal for second-generation Americans; almost everyone speaks it. Since it is not a source of behavioral variation among most American populations (i.e., between families), it is not an environmental influence that is peculiar to a specific family. Second, environmental exposures must be experienced by all siblings. Divorce qualifies here because all siblings within a family experience it, but perinatal traumas, which tend to differ from child to child, do not. Third, the environmental exposure must have a directional effect on a given trait to be considered an environmental influence on that trait. For instance, exposure to radon gas could be a shared environmental influence according to conditions one and two: it is correlated across siblings, yet concentrations of the radioactive gas vary from one household to another. However, radon gas does not have a direct effect on IQ and hence is not a shared environmental influence for IQ. In contrast, radon gas could be a shared environmental risk for later cancers, because exposure to this gas has been directly linked to later mobidity.

Finally, environmental effects can be shared environmental influences only to the extent that they reliably change a trait in a *constant* direction. For example, divorce is correlated across siblings and varies from household to household (conditions 2 and 1, respectively). Thus, divorce may be a shared environmental influence on achievement if it is harmful (or helpful) to most children's academic efforts (condition 3). However, to the extent that children react *differently* to parental divorce (e.g., one child may study diligently to avoid witnessing parental conflicts, whereas a brother or sister may become so disturbed as to be unable to study), the influence of the shared *exposure* to divorce is counted as a nonshared rather than a shared environmental influence.

The second type of environmental effect in behavioral genetic models—nonshared environmental influences—by definition consists of environmental effects that operate to make siblings dissimilar. Many measurable influences may have this kind of effect. For example, accidents of embryological development fall into this class of influence because they differ from one fetus to another. Common nonshared influences include such processes as differential parental treatment, friendships, illnesses and childhood accidents, and perinatal traumas. Influences associated with birth order are also nonshared, because birth order is unique to each child within a family except in the case of twins. Finally, as mentioned earlier, environmental effects that are shared by siblings yet have different effects on their development count as nonshared environmental influences. The number and variety of potential nonshared environmental influences are nearly limitless.

In most statistical models, nonshared environmental influences are easily confounded with measurement error because measurement error also contributes to dissimilarity in family members. For example, the height correlation between monozygotic (identical, or MZ) twins is greater when measurements are done with an accurate tape measure. Measurements taken with a tape that has stretched or shrunk between measurements result in a gross underestimate of the MZ twins' *true* resemblance. Thus, unless estimated and statistically controlled, measurement error variance becomes a component of the nonshared environmental effect in traditional behavioral genetics models.

In addition to the difference between shared and nonshared environmental influences, an important distinction is made in behavioral genetics to reflect the nature of the interrelation between genetics and environment in producing a given behavioral effect. The two types of relationships are called gene → environment (g → e) *correlations* and gene × environment (g × e) *interactions.* G × e interactions occur when phenotypes change dramatically in response to a specific *combination* of environmental and genetic influences. A classic example of a g × e interaction is the metabolic disease phenylketonuria (PKU). Susceptibility is created genetically when a homozygous mutant gene is inherited. The mutant alleles shut down the metabolism of the amino acid phenylalanine, leading to the accumulation of toxic byproducts in the body. However, the disease occurs only when a rare susceptibility—the presence of the homozygous recessive gene—encounters a particular environmental stimulus: an amino acid found in meats and in many other foods. Thus, the disease is avoidable if the person who is at genetic risk is placed on a diet low in phenylalanine. PKU is an example of a g × e interaction because it occurs only when both genetic susceptibility and specific environmental conditions are present; one or the other is not sufficient. G × e interactions are interesting because changes in the "mix" of genetic and environmental conditions result in differences in phenotypes. On the other hand, g × e interactions are rarely found in the behavioral genetics of common traits (see the discussion of interactions in McCall 1991).

G → e correlations are distinct from g × e interactions. G → e correlations capture the empirical evidence that certain phenotypes are significantly associated with specific environments; thus they refer to the *nonrandom* assignment of phenotypes to particular environments. G → e correlations can occur when environments react to a given phenotype, or when those possessing a given phenotype actively seek a certain environment. To the extent that genes partly engineer the phenotype, then genes and environments become correlated. The "halo effect" often found for attractive people illustrates a reactive g → e correlation because genes affect physical appearance which, in turn, elicits either social approval or disapproval.

The active form of the g → e correlation involves the selection of environments that reinforce particular phenotypes. For example, bright children often read more than other children. This creates a g → e correlation between IQ (a phenotype brought about by a combination of genes, shared environmental effects, and nonshared environmental effects) and intellectual stimulation that then furthers the development of intelligence. In this way, genes become correlated with environmental exposures. In behavioral genetic designs, the active and reactive g → e correlations both count in the genetic component of variation—they add to the heritability estimate.

G → e correlations also have a relation to experimental design. The presence of g → e correlations may create methodological confounds because social categories may also be genetic ones. For example, the variable "social class" is often used in family socialization studies as an environmental variable. This assumes that the average genotype for lower-class individuals is the same as that for middle- and upper-class individuals. However, data from twin and adoption studies have invalidated this assumption; there is ample evidence that social class has heritable components, as would be expected from the known differences in heritable traits such as IQ (Herrnstein and Murray 1994; Rowe 1994). Thus, the common practice of equating average genotypes across social classes as a control for environmental group differences is, given these data, unjustified. Other "typical" controls in tests for environmental effects may likewise obscure potential genetic influences.

Current Directions in Behavioral Genetic Research

The modern behavioral genetic model is a blend of different methodological approaches, based primarily on path analysis and analysis of variance techniques that were part of "biometrical genetics" (Neale and Cardon 1992). It is characterized by (1) the use of multiple kinship groups, often more than just MZ and dizygotic (DZ) twin groups; (2) the statement of a path analytic model using pairs of relatives' trait variances and covariances; and (3) the fitting of this model to observations (usually covariance matrices) with structural equation programs (e.g., Mx, *LISREL*) that estimate goodness-of-fit and various genetic and environmental parameters (e.g., heritability).

Behavioral genetic research designs help to identify models that would otherwise be unavailable for use in social science. The concept of model identification is a complex one. To make a simple analogy, given two separate equations with *x* and *y* variables where each variable retains the same value in both equations, one can solve for *x* and *y*. However, given two equations, one with *x*, *y*, and *z* variables and the other with *x* and *y* variables, one cannot solve for *x*, *y*, and *z* because two equations do not give enough information to solve for three unknowns. The first pair of equations is an "identified" model; the second is not. In other words, an identified model makes it possible to assign values to variables. The ability of behavioral genetic designs to "identify" complex models allows for the exploration of many interesting questions about influences on behavior, including how to use data from multiple informants or raters, how to explain behavioral development, and what creates correlation between phenotypes. Although these topics do not exhaust research activity in behavioral genetics, they serve as good illustrations and they are considered in turn in the next sections.

Behavioral Genetic Analysis of Multiple Informants

Consider an interesting problem in explaining trait variation: how to "distill" a trait from various ratings of behavior (Rowe and Kandel, 1997). The multiple raters may have a *shared view* of a target child, based on their observations of behavior. However, each rater may also have an *individual view* of the child, resulting from many influences (e.g., experiences one rater but not the other has had with the child, perceptual biases, and so on). The shared view may be interpreted as the child's generalized or global behavioral trait. Multiple raters are often used to estimate this general trait more accurately. With only a single child and two ratings of behavior, however, there is no way to separate the influence of shared and individual views on raters' judgments.

Figure 1 shows an example of two measures of a phenotype. One is the mother's rating; the other is the child's self-rating. Both measures help to define the child's true trait (path coefficients a and b). However, the mother's rating is also influenced by her individual view (path coefficient c). This model nicely states the sources of variation, but it is not an identified model because there is not enough information to solve for all three path coefficients simultaneously. It can be rescued, however, by putting it into a behavioral genetic research design (i.e., a sibling pair design).

Figure 2 draws the comparable model for sibling pairs. As each mother rates two of her children, her *individual view* is allowed to influence both ratings (path coefficient q). The child's trait influences both the mother's rating (a) and the child's self-rating (b). The path coefficients c and h reflect shared environment and genetic influences, respectively. This model permits two sources of sibling resemblance—one through correlated genes (genetic effects, designated by the path $h x r_g x h$) and the other through shared environments (shared environmental effects, designated by the path $c x 1.0 x c$). Nonshared environmental influences (e) also have an impact on the traits. Although this model is more complex than the model in which each mother rates only one child (as in Figure 1), it is also mathematically identified when covariance matrices are fit for two or more groups (e.g., MZ and DZ twins, or full and half-siblings). Thus, in addition to answering the behavioral genetic question of the estimation of genetic and environmental effects, this model also addresses a question of broad interest to personality researchers: how maternal and child ratings contribute to the estimate of the "true" trait. Neither of these questions could be answered by using the model shown in Figure 1.

As an example, Simonoff et al. (1995) explored a variety of behavioral genetic models of rater effects for rating disruptive behavior in childhood (i.e., 8–16 years) using twin data. Ratings on the twin children's disruptive behavior came from child self-reports, mothers' reports, and fathers' reports. Although their article should be consulted for details, these authors found that genetic effects increased for the *shared view*, that is, for a global trait inferred from multiple ratings, and shared environmental influences decreased (Simonoff et al. 1995, 318).[1] Shared environmental influences decreased because some of the within-parent correlation was explained by the individual view of each

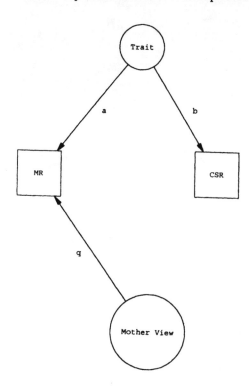

Figure 1. Single child model (MR = mother rating, CSR = child self-rating).

rater. The individual (parental) views were also correlated in the best-fitting model. Parents may agree separately about their children because of shared expectations or other influences that do not relate to a child's global traits. Regardless of the correct explanation of the individual view, it is clear that behavioral genetics offers a method for examining the etiology of a global trait as defined by multiple ratings. In general, in the models of Siminoff et al., a global trait inferred from shared view ratings showed greater genetic influence than behavior associated with individual views.

Behavioral Development

Behavioral development is marked by both stability and change. For example, the stability of self-reports of delinquency fall into the $r = 0.50$–0.70 range

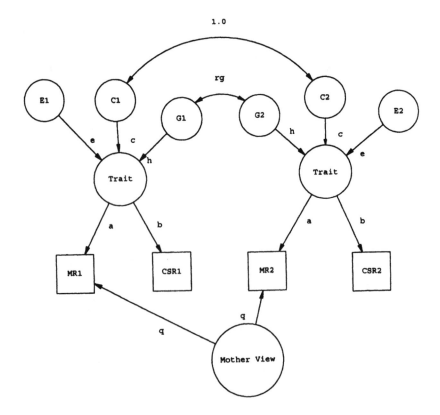

Figure 2. Sibling model (1 designates one sibling, 2 the other sibling, E = nonshared environment, C = shared environment, G = heredity).

across three years of adolescence (Rowe and Britt 1991). Nonetheless, many adolescents who start out as delinquents desist from crime by the end of their teenaged years. This mixed picture of stability and change can be found for many traits. The longitudinal design allows one to examine individuals as they mature, as they both change and stay the same. The strengths of the design for establishing causal order and for examining change are widely understood. However, the contribution of longitudinal studies to advancing theory about environmental and genetic influences on development is less appreciated. Furthermore, although several scholars have enthusiastically promoted developmental behavioral genetics (Plomin 1986; Rutter 1994), there has been limited use of these designs because data that are both longitudinal and kinship based are rare.

Developmental behavioral genetics deals with the determinants of stability and change in behavioral traits. The field combines a longitudinal design with a kinship design; that is, more than one age of measurement for pairs of relatives who differ in their genetic relatedness. Three periods of observation are necessary to mathematically identify (i.e., make solvable) the more complex developmental designs.

Developmental behavioral genetic designs distinguish between two broad classes of developmental mechanisms—transmission and liability or common factors. In the *transmission model*, earlier experiences send their influence forward in time so that successive periods of functioning are causally linked. The idea of transmission is present in many developmental theories. In criminology, labeling theory assumes that arrest or other contact with the justice system changes the self-concept so that the individual is more likely to commit future crimes. Similarly, gang involvement might temporarily increase the likelihood of later criminal offenses. In attachment theory, the security of infant attachment is assumed to create a "mental model" of relationships that may extend to romance in adolescence. Developmental concepts that highlight *critical periods or developmental tasks* claim that outcomes of certain phases affect future functioning.

The transmission model resembles the concept of *state dependence* in demography and sociology. In state dependence, past behavior affects future behavior. For instance, the mere commission of a crime may loosen social commitments toward conventionality so that another crime becomes more probable. State dependence also comes into play as life events occur that may alter an individual's state and thus redirect behavior. In the example of criminal acts, marriage is thought to cause some criminals to desist. As new influences enter and affect behavioral development, change is instigated.

The second class of developmental models can be referred to as *liability* or *common factor* models. In these models, no causal relation between subsequent time points is assumed. In the liability model, the stability of development arises from underlying individual differences, which may be only partly understood. The continuum of these individual differences is called a "liability." This liability may act as a "third variable" that makes the stability of behavior from one age to the next noncausal; temporal order alone does not establish that a prior variable is a cause of one that follows it in time.

The trait of blood pressure can be used to illustrate the liability model. Blood pressure is highly stable over the life course. This stability, however, does not mean that high blood pressure at one age *directly causes* high blood pressure at a later age. Instead, it is more likely that individual differences in physiology—some of which are targeted by blood pressure medications— make some people prone to life-long high blood pressure. Liability mechanisms can also account for change, because at each point in time there may be new effects of other variables, such as the introduction of medicines, which might cause changes in blood pressure. The essential assumption, however, is that continuity is completely explained by the underlying liability, not by previous scores on a trait or behavior.

In demography and criminology, the liability model sometimes goes under the name of *heterogeneity*. Heterogeneity refers to all sources of individual differences that are not directly measured in a research design. The known covariates, of course, can be used in regression analyses as statistical controls, and their effects on other variables partialled away, but unknown covariates cannot be controlled for and remain as validity threats. For example, divorced and nondivorced groups may be matched for social class, but such matching might leave personality differences uncontrolled. One advantage of a developmental genetic design is that the liability can be treated as a latent variable that includes the influences of all sources of heterogeneity, whether measured or not.

Both the transmission and liability models assume a certain amount of developmental stability. These models, however, imply rather different patterns of stability among assessments in a longitudinal study. In the transmission model, assessments closer in time should be more highly correlated than more distant ones. This "autoregressive" pattern occurs because, while the effects of prior experiences are felt for some time, new experiences and events also enter the developmental process and can create change. For example, suppose we have data on self-reported delinquency from assessments at three ages that yielded these correlations: $r_{12} = 0.55$, $r_{23} = 0.55$, and $r_{13} = 0.30$. The most separated assessments (r_{13}) show the lowest stability correlation; furthermore, as expected under an autoregressive process, the stability from the first to the last assessment exactly equals the product of the correlations between adjacent assessments (i.e., $0.30 = 0.55 \times 0.55$). This hypothetical example also demonstrates the need for assessments from three or more time periods, because two assessments provide no test of this autoregressive property. In contrast, the liability model assumes that the same stable mechanisms exert their effects at each assessment and does not imply a decrease in stability with an increase of the time lag between assessments. In a pure liability model, stability from the first to the third assessment of delinquency would be 0.55, the same as the correlations between adjacent time points.

The goodness-of-fit of liability and transmission models can be compared using behavioral genetic designs. For example, Van den Oord and Rowe (1997) looked at the stability of problem behaviors in children assessed at three ages: 4–6 years, 6–8 years, and 8–10 years. The measure of problem behavior was a maternal checklist of problem behaviors, where items were rated as "often true," "sometimes true," and "not true" of a child. The children were either siblings or cousins, and the children who were siblings were either full or maternal half-siblings. These three groups were used to fit both liability and transmission models that estimated behavioral genetic parameters. On the whole, the liability model performed substantially better than the transmission model. The liability model did not require time-specific effects, and it showed that the combination of a genetic liability and a shared environmental liability together accounted for the stability of problem behaviors from 4 to 10 years. Thus, results from this study suggest that previous problem behavior does not cause later problem behavior; rather, stable genetic and environmental factors influence problem behavior at each of the three time points. In addition, the study also revealed that the largest contribution to age-related *change* in problem behavior was due to nonshared environmental influences. In summary, developmental behavioral genetic methods examine genetic, shared environmental, and nonshared environmental mechanisms underlying age-to-age continuity and change (see Eaves et al. 1986; Hewitt et al. 1988; Philips and Fulker 1989).

Genetic and Environmental Mediators of
Covariances and Correlations

Perhaps the most common use of behavioral genetic designs is apportioning covariance between phenotypes to genetic and environmental sources of variation. Many questions about causality depend on the source of variation between two phenotypes. Analysis of the covariance or correlation between phenotypes may be bivariate when just two variables are involved, or may involve complex multivariate models (e.g., psychometric and biometric models, see Neale and Cardon 1992). For example, traits X and Y may be correlated within individuals. Now, if both traits are heritable, then their correlation might arise because of a genetic correlation between them. That is, genes that affect more than one phenotype can produce a genetic correlation (technically, *pleiotropy*). As an illustration, consider that the gene for albino skin coloration in mice also produces behavioral inhibition in an open field test (Plomin et al. 1997). Thus, coat color and behavioral inhibition are correlated traits in mice because they are partly caused by the same gene.

Sources of covariance can also be environmental. Shared environmental influences common to two or more phenotypes may induce correlation between them. For example, in adolescence, shared environments (e.g., parental beliefs) influence social attitudes (Eaves et al. 1997). The covariance typically found among different attitudes tends to occur because some parental beliefs influence more than one attitude. As an adolescent models parental beliefs, he accepts the same "suite" of attitudes as the parent; thus a shared environmental effect on the covariance among attitudes occurs. It is interesting that the effects of shared family environments on social attitudes sharply diminish once the adolescent leaves home and enters the working world; at the same time, the heritability (i.e., the genetic influence) of social attitudes increases.

Nonshared environmental influences are also a potential source of covariance among phenotypes *within* an individual. However, nonshared environmental effects, as noted earlier in this chapter, are unique to each individual and thus always reduce the behavioral resemblance *between* family members. For example, some part of the correlation of height and weight within an individual is explained by common genes that influence body size. However, another part of this within-person correlation may arise from nonshared environmental influences on body size, including almost accidental aspects of embryological development, or factors such as nutrition, which might vary *across* individuals.

The analysis of covariance has many uses. Two examples illustrate two extremely different applications, one analyzing the physiological substrates of traits, the other analyzing their environmental correlates. Although heritability implies the existence of a physiological substrate for a trait, the phenotypic association between a trait and a biological marker for it is not sufficient proof of a common genetic effect. Better early nutrition, for example, may increase both body and brain size. If so, a correlation between brain size and IQ could be mediated by environmental influences (both shared and nonshared) related to nutrition, rather than by genetic influences.

Another physical variable that has a phenotypic association with IQ—nerve conduction velocity—has been analyzed in a twin study (Rijsdik and Boomsma 1997). Nerve conduction velocity is measured in peripheral nerves in the arm and reflects the speed with which nerve impulses move through axons and across synapses. In this twin sample, conduction velocity and IQ had a correlation of 0.20. The bivariate analysis of this within-person correlation revealed that the association between IQ and nerve conduction velocity was entirely genetic. Thus, the same genes that influence conduction velocity also influence IQ, and the former is a good physiological marker for individual differences in IQ that are due to genes.

The second type of bivariate analysis deals with the association of children's traits and environmental measures. A typical interpretation of the association is that it is causal; that is to say, the environmental influences causally affect the trait. This interpretation suggests that a decomposition of the association between shared environmental influences (such as parental treatment) and children's traits involves the environmental influences only and not genetic influences. However, another possibility is that the decomposition involves genetic effects alone. This situation could arise if genes in a parent affect parental behaviors related to childrearing *and* if copies of those same genes, expressed in the children, produce the behavioral trait that is the dependent variable of interest. A causal association between parental treatment and children's behavior, then, would be spurious (i.e., noncausal) because genes, not environmental effects, create it.

An example of a study examining the relationship between children's traits and environmental measures is the bivariate genetic analysis of the relationship between parental negativity and adolescent antisocial behavior carried out by Pike et al. (Pike et al. 1996). The genetically informative groups consisted of MZ twins, DZ twins, full siblings, half-siblings, and biologically unrelated siblings. Parental negativity was measured by parental self-reports and observations of parent-child interactions. Antisocial behavior was measured by the children's (10–18 years of age) self-report of antisocial acts and by the extent to which the adolescents were disruptive or disrespectful during home observations of them.

It is possible to anticipate the findings of Pike et al.'s more complex model fitting by examining the cross-correlations between siblings. A sibling correlation is simply trait X on sibling 1 correlated with trait X on sibling 2, whereas a sibling cross-correlation is trait X on sibling 1 correlated with trait Y on sibling 2 (or vice versa). In this study, the sibling cross-correlation is the parental negativity directed toward sibling 1 correlated with sibling 2's antisocial behavior (and vice versa). To the extent that genetic influences are important, cross-correlations should increase in step with the genetic relatedness of each sibling group. In Pike et al.'s study, the correlations of the mother's negativity toward sibling 1 and the antisocial behavior of sibling 2 were MZ twins, 0.54; DZ twins, 0.34; full siblings, 0.30; half-siblings, 0.34; and unrelated siblings, 0.18. Although the half-siblings are more alike than the genetic expectation, as are the unrelated siblings reared together, the pattern of cross-correlations clearly suggests a genetic effect.

This genetic effect was also borne out by the results of Pike et al.'s model fitting. The phenotypic correlation between negativity and antisocial behavior ($r = 0.60$) was apportioned to genetic influence (0.40), shared environment (0.16), and nonshared environment (0.05). In other words, 66 percent of the total association between parent negativity and child antisocial behavior was mediated genetically (i.e., 0.40/0.60). Two explanations can be offered for this genetic mediation. One is that negativity in a parent is simply another expression of antisocial behavior, so that the same genetic trait surfaces differently, depending on age and social role (i.e., antisocial behavior in adolescents vs. negative parenting in adults). Adolescents, who usually have no children of their own, lack the opportunity to display their antisocial behavior in terms of poor parenting behaviors. On the other hand, parental treatment also differs from sibling to sibling. This favors a different explanation: namely, that a child's heritable antisocial behavior partly elicits negativity from a parent (see also Ge et al. 1996; McGue et al. 1996). In both explanations, however, the commonplace view that an association between parental behavior and child outcome can be interpreted as solely environmental in origin must be abandoned.

G × e Interactions

As mentioned earlier, surprisingly few g × e interactions are found in behavioral genetic research. In most cases, additive models, which do not allow for g × e interactions, fit data extremely well (Rowe 1994). There are a few cases of g × e interactions (Eaves et al. 1997). In one case, the relative importance of genetic and shared environmental influences on social attitudes was found to shift with age. In adolescence, shared environmental influences dominate the total variation. For example, in the mid-teens, both MZ and DZ twin correlations of social attitudes fell into the range 0.40–0.60. A genetic effect would show up in a greater MZ twin correlation; thus it would appear as though genetics has little influence on the social attitudes of adolescents. In contrast, the presence of a significant correlation between twins suggests some shared environmental influence. After age 20, however, the twin correlations strikingly diverged. The MZ twin correlation settled to a value of about 0.70 and the DZ twin correlation to about 0.40. In other words, in one environment (i.e., adolescents living together in their home), the genes relevant to social attitudes were not expressed. However, in the environment of adult life, when twins usually live apart from one another, enter the workforce, and make individual political choices that might increase the relevance of their social attitudes, social attitudes become genetically influenced.

In another case of g × e interaction, Rowe et al. (in press) explored the magnitude of genetic and environmental influences on adolescent verbal IQ for different levels of parental education. The overall heritability of verbal IQ was about 0.55. The heritability was significantly greater among more well-educated familes. In contrast, however, at lower levels of parental education (i.e., less than high school), shared environmental effects increased. Thus, shared environmental influences varied from about zero in well-educated families to 28 percent of the total variation in poorly educated families. One explanation for this pattern is that intellectual stimulation may be widely available in the *nonfamily* environments of well-educated children, such as through their schools and peer groups. Thus, a child from a well-educated family that provides low intellectual stimulation can compensate by finding intellectual stimulation outside the home. In contrast, a child from a poorly educated family may not have this opportunity, or it may be less available. Thus, in a neighborhood of better-educated families, the particular level of stimulation *within* families becomes less important, reducing the shared environmental effect to nil.

Overall, the general absence of many g × e interactions is noteworthy, yet an absence of replicable interaction effects is not new in social science. For example, Cronbach and Snow (1975) concluded that aptitude x treatment interactions were rare. The absence of interactions in behavioral genetics may partly reflect the great technical demands needed to uncover them, such as the need for large samples and the relative rarity of the genotypes or environments most productive of interaction effects (McClelland and Judd 1993). However, McCall (1991) suggests a more profound reason for the relative absence of interactions: Nature may avoid interactions because the dependence of development on particular environmental circumstances is maladaptive. If the successful development of a trait were to become too tightly constrained by environmental influences, it would be exposed to the "struggle for existence" of natural selection, and would tend to result in death, and thereby the loss of the particular gene (or genes) from the population. Whatever the reason, the general absence of interactions has been one of the more unexpected findings of behavioral genetic research.

The Shared Environment Controversy

Finally, it is ironic that the most startling finding of behavioral genetics since 1945 has not been a discovery about *genetic* influences (i.e., heritability), but rather a discovery about *shared environmental* effects. The main finding has been that shared environmental effects are negligible for most behavioral traits (and for many physical ones as well). Because this finding threatens the core assumptions of several disciplines, it has aroused as much controversy as the earlier—but now widely accepted—conclusion that behavioral traits are at least in part heritable (Baumrind 1993; Brody 1995; Eaves et al. 1989; Jackson 1993; Lerner 1995; Rende 1995; Rowe 1995; Scarr 1992, 1993; Wachs 1995).

As summarized by Rowe (1994), most behavioral genetic studies, using a variety of methods (e.g., twin, adoption, and family studies) find negligible shared environmental effects. Shared environmental effects, as defined above, arise from exposures to environmental influences *common* to siblings. An absence of shared effects could have two causes. One is that a particular shared influence simply has no effect, as is the case in one example cited at the beginning of this chapter: shared exposure to radon gas fails to influence IQ. The other reason for the absence of shared environmental effects is that exposure to similar environments may have unpredictable effects from one sibling to another. In another example used earlier in this chapter, divorce may disrupt the academic efforts of one sibling but encourage those of another (who may retreat to the books to avoid emotional conflict). In either case, the negligible shared environmental effect is dismaying for those who believe that interventions aimed at parental treatments and more general aspects of family environment such as income and parental education can reliably change the trait outcomes for children in a *favorable* direction. However, it should be noted that the absence of shared environmental influences does *not* deny that children react to the parental treatments—they do. However, their reactions do not seem to be unidirectional, so that a particular family milieu will not *reliably* produce a particular trait. Furthermore, the shy child, the aggressive child, and the low-IQ child seem to acquire their traits from a combination of *nonshared* environmental influences and heredity (which parents, of course, provide but do not control). These findings are broadly important for social interventions aimed at changing parental behaviors because they suggest that many of these interventions will fail. In light of this knowledge, then, there is a need to move the importance of global family environmental influences downward, and to integrate this knowledge into our theories of behavioral development.

Conclusion and Retrospect

Behavioral genetics is now part of the mainstream of social science, particularly in the disciplines of psychology and psychiatry. Its ideas, findings, and methods have been increasingly adopted throughout social science. The field is producing data on the role of genetic and environmental influences on behavioral development, on the associations between parental treatment and child outcomes, and on the biological markers related to traits. Finally, in its ability to separate and identify genetic and environmental influences on behavior, behavioral genetics is also revolutionizing our understanding of how environmental influences work. These scientific advances make it essential that scholars who are interested in behavioral development become familiar with findings and methods in behavioral genetics. Scarr's "three cheers" for behavioral genetics should probably be reserved for the time when this field is fully integrated with other fields, including sociology and cultural anthropology. At the pace social science is now moving, this integration may be close at hand.

Note

1. Our use of "shared view" is different from that of Simonoff et al., who use the term to refer to the correlation of the mother's and father's view rather than to the loadings of ratings on the global trait. The reader should be alert to this change in vocabulary.

References

Baumrind, D. 1993. The average expectable environment is not good enough: A response to Scarr. *Child Dev.* 64: 1299–1377.

Brody, N. 1995. Beyond family influences. *Psychol. Inquiry* 6: 142–145.

Cronbach, L. J., and R. E. Snow. 1975. *Aptitudes and Instructional Methods: A Handbook for Research on Intervention.* New York: Irvington.

Crow, J. F. 1993. Francis Galton: Count and measure, measure and count. *Genetics* 135: 1–4.

Degler, C. N. 1991. *In Search of Human Nature: The Decline and Revival of Darwinism in American Social Thought.* New York: Oxford University Press.

Eaves, L. J., J. Long, and A. C. Heath. 1986. A theory of developmental change in quantitative phenotypes applied to cognitive development. *Behav. Genet.* 16: 143–162.

Eaves, L. J., H. J. Eysenck, and N. G. Martin. 1989. *Genes, Culture and Personality: An Empirical Approach.* London: Academic Press.

Eaves, L., N. Martin, A. Heath, et al. 1997. Age changes in the causes of individual differences in conservatism. *Behav. Genet.* 27: 121–124.

Fisher, R. A. 1918. The correlation between relatives on the supposition of Mendelian inheritance. *Trans. R. Soc. Edinb.* 52: 399–433.

Ge, X., R. D. Conger, R. I. Cadoret, et al. 1996. The developmental interface between nature and nurture: A mutual influence model of child antisocial behavior and parent behavior. *Dev. Psychol.* 32: 574–589.

Herrnstein, R. J., and C. Murray. 1994. *The Bell Curve: Intelligence and Class Structure in American Life.* New York: Free Press.

Heston, L. L. 1966. Psychiatric disorders in foster home reared children of schizophrenic mothers. *Br. J. Psychiatry* 112: 819–825.

Hewitt, J. K., L. J. Eaves, M. C. Neale, and J. M. Meyer. 1988. Resolving causes of developmental continuity or "tracking." I: Longitudinal twin studies during growth. *Behav. Genet.* 18: 133–151.

Jackson, J. F. 1993. Human behavioral genetics, Scarr's theory, and her views on interventions: A critical review and commentary on their implications for African American families. *Child Dev.* 64: 1318–1332.

Kuhn, T. S. 1962. *The Structure of Scientific Revolutions.* Chicago: University of Chicago Press.

Lerner, R. M. 1995. The limits of biological influence: Behavioral genetics as the emperor's new clothes. *Psychol. Inquiry* 6: 145–156.

Neale, M. C., and L. R. Cardon. 1992. *Methodology for Genetic Studies of Twins and Families.* Dordrecht, the Netherlands: Kluwer Academic.

McCall, R. 1991. So many interactions, so little evidence. Why? In *Conceptualization and Measurement of Organism-Environment Interaction,* T. D. Wachs and R. Plomin, eds., 146–161. Washington, D.C.: American Psychological Association.

McClelland, G. H., and C. M. Judd. 1993. Statistical difficulties of detecting interactions and moderator effects. *Psychol. Bull.* 114: 376–390.

McGue, M., A. Sharma, and P. Benson. 1996. The effect of common rearing on adolescent adjustment: Evidence from a U.S. adoption cohort. *Dev. Psychol.* 32: 604–613.

Philips, K. I., and D. W. Fulker. 1989. Quantitative genetic analysis of longitudinal trends in adoption designs with application to IQ in the Colorado Adoption Project. *Behav. Genet.* 19: 621–658.

Pike, A., S. McGuire, E. M. Hetherington, D. Reiss, and R. Plomin. 1996. Family environment and adolescent depressive symptoms and antisocial behavior: A multivariate genetic analysis. *Dev. Psychol.* 32: 590–603.

Plomin, R. 1986. *Development, Genetics, and Psychology.* Hillsdale, N.J.: Erlbaum.

Plomin, R., J. C. DeFries, G. E. McClearn, and M. Rutter. 1997. *Behavioral Genetics,* 3d ed. New York: Freeman.

Reiss, D. 1995. Genetic influence on family systems: Implications for development. *J. Marriage Family* 57: 543–560.

Rende, R. 1995. The limits of genetic influences: A new horizon for behavior genetics. *Psychol. Inquiry* 6: 157–160.

Rijsdik, F. V., and D. I. Boomsma. 1997. Genetic mediation of the correlation between peripheral nerve conduction velocity and IQ. *Behav. Genet.* 27: 87–98.

Rowe, D. C. 1994. *The Limits of Family Influence: Genes, Experience, and Behavior.* New York: Guilford.

Rowe, D. C. 1995. The limits of family influence: A response. *Psychol. Inquiry* 6: 174–182.

Rowe, D. C., and C. L. Britt. 1991. Developmental explanations of delinquent behavior among siblings: Common factor vs. transmission. *J. Quant. Criminol.* 7: 315–332.

Rowe, D. C., K. C. Jacobson, and E. J. C. G. Van den Oord. In press. Genetic and environmental influences on vocabulary IQ: Parental education as moderator. *Child Development.*

Rowe, D. C., and D. Kandel. 1997. In the eye of the beholder? Parental ratings of externalizing and internalizing symptoms. *J. Abnorm. Child Psychol.* 25: 265–275.

Rutter, M. 1994. Beyond longitudinal data: Causes, consequences, changes and continuity. *J. Consult. Clin. Psychol.* 62: 928–940.

Scarr, S. 1987. Three cheers for behavior genetics: Winning the war and losing our identity. *Behav. Genet.* 17: 219–228.

Scarr, S. 1992. Developmental theories for the 1990s: Development and individual differences. *Child Dev.* 63: 1–19.

Scarr, S. 1993. Biological and cultural diversity: The legacy of Darwin for development. *Child Dev.* 64: 1333–1353.

Simonoff, E., A. Pickles, J. Hewitt, et al. 1995. Multiple raters of disruptive child behavior: Using a genetic strategy to examine shared views and bias. *Behav. Genet.* 25: 311–326.

Van den Oord, E. J. C. G., and D. C. Rowe. 1997. Continuity and change in children's maladjustment: A developmental behavior genetic study. *Dev. Psychol.* 33: 319–332.

Wachs, T. D. 1995. Genetic and family influences on individual development: Both necessary, neither sufficient. *Psychol. Inquiry* 6: 161–173.

3 Identifying the Molecular Genetic Basis of Behavioral Traits

Stephanie L. Sherman, Ph.D. and
Irwin D. Waldman, Ph.D.

There has been no better time to be a researcher in the field of human genetics. Although positions as a collaborator of Gregor Mendel or of Watson and Crick may have held similar charms, never has research in human genetics had a greater armamentarium. The number of identified and cloned genes has been growing at an exponential rate, so that the whole human genome should be sequenced by 2005. "High-tech" laboratory techniques such as polymerase chain reaction (PCR) have made it possible to genotype many loci from only a small initial quantity of DNA, allowing "low-tech" procedures for the collection of DNA in as unobtrusive a manner as imaginable (e.g., buccal brushes). Statistical developments are enabling human genetics researchers to locate genes and quantify their effects on both diseases and "normal-range" traits in more effective and efficient ways. It is little wonder that a month does not pass without some dramatic new finding in human genetics.

For a variety of reasons, the promise of interesting new findings has been actualized to a much greater extent for the genetics of medical diseases than for the genetics of psychiatric disorders or behavioral traits, although the recent advances mentioned above are just as pertinent for both fields. While the major genes underlying diseases such as Huntington disease, cystic fibrosis, Duchenne muscular dystrophy, and breast cancer have been located and cloned, a succession of initial positive findings and subsequent failures to replicate those findings have been reported for psychiatric disorders, including schizophrenia, bipolar disorder, and Tourette syndrome.

Why the recurrent disappointments for psychiatric disorders? A number of reasons come readily to mind. First, many issues in the accuracy and validity of the classification of psychiatric disorders remain to be resolved. Although the classification and diagnosis of medical diseases are continually evolving, they are at a much more advanced stage than those for their psychiatric counterparts. Second, as a corollary of these issues in classification and diagnosis, it is likely that genetic influences of psychiatric disorders act at the level of component traits rather than at the level of the disorders per se. For example, specific genes that influence schizophrenia are more likely to affect its component symptoms or symptom dimensions such as thought disorder, flat affect and anhedonia, attentional dysfunction, and hallucinations, than to act at the level of the overall disorder. Hence, searches for specific genes for psychiatric disorders per se may not be as fruitful as searches for genes that influence specific symptom dimensions of these disorders. Third, it has been suggested that there may be genetic heterogeneity for psychiatric disorders, both in the sense of independent genetic influences for a particular disorder and in the sense that different genes may affect distinct subtypes of disorders. Fourth, psychiatric disorders and behavioral traits may best be construed as "complex traits" from a genetic standpoint, making them more like diabetes and cardiovascular disease than Huntington disease and cystic fibrosis. That is, such traits are not inherited in a simple Mendelian pattern, but most likely are due to the effects of many genes, each playing a weak role in the development of the trait. The issues involved in finding genes for complex traits are formidable and are described later in this chapter. In our opinion, it is likely that new statistical genetic methods for complex traits will be needed to find genes for psychiatric disorders and behavioral traits. The purpose of this chapter is to describe some of these methods for finding genes for complex traits, as well as to present some examples of recent successes in the domains of psychiatric disorders and behavioral traits.

From Statistical Estimates of Genetic Influences to the Effects of Specific Genes

A useful preliminary stage to molecular genetic studies is the use of behavioral genetic studies to disentangle and characterize genetic and environmental influences. (These methods are described in more detail in Chapter 2 in this volume.) Behavioral genetic studies are useful in quantifying the magnitude of genetic and environmental influences, albeit in a broad, statistical manner through abstract variance components. In addition, although family studies determine the extent to which a trait or disorder clusters in families, twin and adoption studies are necessary in order to disentangle genetic from environmental influences and to estimate the magnitude of each. Twin studies have certain advantages over adoption studies, including (1) ease of sampling,

(2) measurement of a trait or disorder contemporaneously in relatives (i.e., twins) rather than relying on the retrospective reports of some relatives (e.g., adoptive parents), and (3) control for many potential confounding variables (e.g., socioeconomic status [SES], ethnicity, neighborhood characteristics) because twins grow up together in the same home.

A brief description of the use of data from twins to estimate genetic and environmental influences may be helpful. Behavioral geneticists typically are interested in disentangling three sets of influences that may cause individual differences or variation in a given trait. First, heritability, or h^2, refers to the proportion of variance in the trait that is due to genetic differences among individuals in the population. Second, shared environmental influences, or c^2, refer to the proportion of variance in the trait that is due to environmental influences that family members experience in common and that increase their similarity for the trait. Third, nonshared environmental influences, or e^2, refer to the proportion of variance in the trait that is due to environmental influences that are experienced uniquely by family members and that decrease their similarity for the trait. To estimate these influences, twin studies rely on the fact that identical or monozygotic (MZ) twins are identical genetically (barring exceptions such as somatic mutations) whereas fraternal or dizygotic (DZ) twins, just like nontwin siblings, are on average only 50 percent genetically similar. It also is assumed that environmental influences on the trait of interest are shared between members of fraternal twin pairs as they are between members of identical twin pairs. Given these assumptions, the correlation between identical twins consists of heritability and shared environmental influences (i.e., $r_{MZ} = h^2 + c^2$), because these are the two sets of influences that can contribute to trait similarity in identical twins. In contrast, the correlation between fraternal twins consists of only one-half of heritability but the same shared environmental influences (i.e., $r_{DZ} = 1/2h^2 + c^2$), reflecting the smaller degree of genetic similarity between fraternal twins. Algebraic manipulation of the two equations for twin similarity allows one to estimate h^2, c^2, and e^2 (viz., $h^2 = 2 [r_{MZ} - r_{DZ}]$, $c^2 = 2r_{DZ} - r_{MZ}$, $e^2 = 1 - r_{MZ}$). Although these influences using twin correlations can be estimated by hand, contemporary behavioral geneticists use biometric model-fitting analytic methods (Neale and Cardon 1992) that make use of additional information on familial relationships (e.g., correlations on nontwin siblings or parents and their children), provide statistical tests of the adequacy of these three influences in accounting for the observed familial correlations, and test alternative models for the causal influences underlying the trait (e.g., a model including genetic and nonshared environmental influences versus a model that also includes shared environmental influences). In addition, regression-based methods have been developed (DeFries and Fulker 1985, 1988) for analyzing data from selected samples, such as probands with a disorder and their co-twins. These methods provide an estimate of the heritability of extreme status on the trait (h_g^2), as well as the difference in the magnitude of heritability for extreme status from that of heritability for normal range variation (viz., $h_g^2 - h^2$).

The detection of genetic influences in a twin study is a useful prelude to molecular genetic analyses for a number of reasons. First, it ensures that there are some genetic influences on a psychiatric disorder or behavioral trait to detect. Second, the magnitude of genetic influences, substantial or small, can guide the approach that molecular geneticists take to find one or multiple genes. Third, differential heritability for subtypes of a disorder also can help refine the search for specific genes. Fourth, once a trait gene is identified, the proportion of the overall magnitude of genetic influences explained by that candidate gene can be quantified using a twin study design.

The Complexities of Finding Genes for Complex Traits

As suggested above, like many medical diseases, virtually all psychiatric disorders and behavioral traits can be considered complex traits from a genetic perspective. Given their non-Mendelian transmission pattern, the lack of a simple one-to-one genotype-phenotype relationship, reduced penetrance of any putative liability-increasing alleles, and the presence of phenocopies, psychiatric disorders and behavioral traits must be approached using contemporary molecular genetic analytic methods.

There are basically four approaches currently used to find genes involved in complex traits: linkage analysis, allele-sharing methods, linkage disequilibrium methods, and experimental crosses using animal systems. All depend on the co-segregation of the trait with some genetic marker of known location, be it an anonymous piece of DNA or a gene of known function. The putative trait gene and the genetic marker will be transmitted together from parent to child when they lie close together on the chromosome (i.e., are "linked"), so close that recombination does not often separate them. Recombination is a natural process that occurs during meiosis and causes genetic material to be exchanged between the maternally and paternally derived chromosomes of a ho-mologous pair. The closer together two genetic markers are, the smaller the chance that recombination will occur between them. A measure of the genetic distance between two markers and/or genes is related to the recombination fraction, or the proportion of meioses in which recombination between the two markers would occur.

When genetic markers are close together (i.e., tightly linked), or perhaps part of the same gene, the probability of recombination is negligible and char-acteristics of the surrounding DNA (i.e., the allele polymorphisms) will be pre-served from generation to generation. This phenomenon of the association of specific alleles of a genetic marker with the trait is called *linkage disequilibrium.*

Each of the four analytic approaches has been used with some success to identify genes involved in complex behavioral traits, such as psychiatric disor-ders. The success of such searches depends on the magnitude of the gene's ef-fect on the behavioral trait; namely, the larger the effect size, the easier the de-tection. The ability to correctly identify the mode of inheritance dictates which approach will be most successful. The basis of the four approaches will be de-scribed in a way similar to that of Lander and Schork (1994), followed by a consideration of strategies that may increase the ability to identify genes and issues of statistical significance.

Linkage Analysis: A Model-Based Approach to Examine Co-segregation

Linkage analysis is a model-based, parametric approach to examining co-segregation of a disorder or trait and a genetic marker. The basic method in-volves developing a model to explain the inheritance pattern of the trait and its possible co-segregation with a specific genetic marker of known location. A comparison of the likelihood of the family data assuming linkage between the susceptibility gene and the marker (M_L) with that assuming no linkage (M_0) provides evidence of whether the putative gene is located in that region of the chromosome. The support for linkage is usually represented by the likelihood ratios, $LR = L([\text{Data } I\,(M_L)]/\,L[\text{Data } I\,(M_0)]$, or the so-called lod score, $Z = \log_{10}(LR)$. The linkage of a trait to a specific marker is suggested if the maxi-mum lod score, Z, exceeds some critical statistical threshold.

This approach is the method of choice when the underlying genetic struc-ture of the trait (e.g., the number of genes involved, the mode of inheritance, penetrance, phenocopy rate) has been well established; hence, it is a powerful method for simple Mendelian traits. For example, this approach was used to identify the linkage between the gene for monoamine oxidase type A (MAOA) and a type of aggressive behavior (Brunner et al. 1993). Linkage analysis was also used to identify the location of the gene for the fragile X syndrome, a type of mental retardation that includes behavioral problems (Verkerk et al. 1991). However, applications to complex, non-Mendelian behavioral traits are problematic because the underlying genetic model is not known. If the genetic model is incorrect, the power to detect linkage is significantly reduced and sometimes may lead to false linkages. Well-known examples of such complications can be cited for several psychiatric disorders, including schizophrenia and manic-depressive disorder (Baron et al. 1987, 1993; Egeland et al. 1987; Kelsoe et al. 1989; Kennedy 1988; Sherrington et al. 1988).

At a minimum, the proposed model must include parameters to specify the genetic component of the trait, including the probability of gene transmission, disease allele frequencies, and penetrance functions. Estimates for some parameters may be known from previous segregation studies (e.g., penetrance and allele frequencies), but most are unknown. Unknown parameters usually are considered nuisance parameters and are sometimes estimated using maximum likelihood. Alternatively, several single major gene effect models can be surveyed by fixing the set of genetic parameters to determine their influence on the linkage result (e.g., Straub et al. 1995).

The consequence of incorrectly specifying the genetic model can be illustrated by examining the effect of misspecifying one parameter of a genetic model, penetrance. Penetrance, or the conditional probability of expressing the trait given a genotype at the disease locus, plays a role in defining the probability of the carrier status of normal individuals in the pedigree. If penetrance is fixed to be higher than the true value, the relative probability for a phenotypically normal individual being a noncarrier will be higher than the alternative (i.e., a carrier with no expression). Under this circumstance, the recombination fraction most likely will be overestimated and linkage to a marker may be missed. If penetrance is fixed too low, the carrier status of normal individuals becomes unknown and the power of the analysis is reduced, although the estimate of the recombination fraction should not be affected. One strategy that is commonly used is to set the penetrance of the disease genotype to almost zero, and thereby use only information from affected family members. This approach will prevent missing a true linkage, although the power of the study is reduced.

Newer methods have been developed to account for more complex patterns of inheritance and linkage to a specific marker (e.g., Amos et al. 1996; Weeks and Lathrop 1995). For example, Bonney (1986) devised a statistical framework to combine segregation and linkage analyses. His regressive models account for familial correlations in the presence of a major gene and other sources of familial correlation. When all sources of familial correlations are taken into account, the power to detect linkage of a complex trait to a marker increases. These and other methodological improvements may increase the possibility of successfully using this type of parametric linkage approach to identify behavioral trait genes.

Allele-Sharing Methods: A Nonparametric Approach to Examining Co-segregation

Allele-sharing methods have the advantage of being model-free (i.e., nonparametric). The null hypothesis states that there is no linkage between the trait and the genetic marker; thus alleles of a genetic marker should follow the expected Mendelian inheritance pattern among affected relative pairs. Evidence for linkage is obtained when affected relatives share the same alleles from a common ancestor (i.e., alleles are identical by descent [IBD]) more often than expected. For example, if a marker is not linked to a disease trait, two affected siblings are expected to share 0, 1, or 2 alleles IBD with frequencies of 25, 50, and 25 percent, respectively. The observed data can be compared with the expected frequencies using a simple χ^2 test. For complex traits, allele-sharing methods are more robust than linkage methods because they are model free. That is, increased sharing of marker alleles among affected relatives will be present irrespective of the mode of inheritance, value of penetrance, phenocopies, multiple disease loci, etc. Nonetheless, such methods are less powerful than linkage analysis when the model can be correctly specified.

Allele-sharing methods depend on the ability to determine if an allele that is shared by two relatives is from the same ancestor (IBD) or possibly from different ancestors but of the same form or state (identical by state [IBS]). Many times genotyping of other relatives (e.g., parents of affected sibling pairs) can provide the information needed to make this distinction. Also, IBD can be inferred from IBS when highly polymorphic markers are used or simultaneous examination of several markers is possible. When this is not possible or data are sparse, other analytical approaches can be used to distinguish IBD from IBS (e.g., Amos et al. 1990; Kruglyak and Lander 1995).

Alternative methods are based on the explicit examination of IBS, ignoring IBD. The affected pedigree member (APM) method of linkage analysis measures the marker similarity between affected individuals in terms of IBS (Weeks and Lange 1988). Methods based on IBS are usually less powerful than those based on IBD. However, the APM method may be useful for late-onset diseases or genome scans because it requires genotyping only affected individuals. The drawback of methods that assess IBS is that they use marker allele frequencies to determine the expected amount of sharing among relatives and thus are sensitive to their estimates. The APM method has proved to be an important tool when it is used in concert with model-based methods to show if evidence is dependent on the specified model. It has been applied to such behavioral disorders as Alzheimer disease (Pericak-Vance et al. 1991) and schizophrenia (Wang et al. 1995).

Allele-sharing methods also can be used for quantitative traits. The basic premise is that the greater the number of alleles shared in common at the putative locus, the more similar the phenotype of two relatives. This can be stated in terms of the regression analysis that is usually applied: the square of the difference in the trait measurement between two relatives should be negatively correlated with the number of alleles shared at the disease-causing locus (Haseman and Elston 1972). Since this is a regression-based method, it can be easily applied to multivariate phenotypes and can incorporate adjustments for covariates.

Since sampling sibling pairs is practical, the properties of allele-sharing approaches for detecting linkage with quantitative traits have been studied most extensively with sibling pairs. Random selection of sibling pairs for linkage studies has been compared with other schemes, including selection of only those with extremes of the phenotype distribution or selection of those who are highly discordant or highly concordant (e.g., Risch and Zhang 1995). Such schemes reduce the number of sibling pairs needed to detect linkage. They also reduce the number of genotypes to be determined, although the number of pairs to be assessed phenotypically remains large, sometimes larger than in a random selection scheme.

Nonparametric Methods for Association and Linkage Disequilibrium

The traditional method of examining the association between a candidate gene and a disease is the case-control method, in which the frequency of a "high-risk" allele among individuals affected with the disease is contrasted with that among individuals without the disease. This latter group could consist of individuals randomly selected from the population or individuals who were matched to cases on a host of potential background confounding variables (e.g., ethnicity, SES, age, gender). In fact, the evolution of case-control methods in the epidemiological literature has focused on the development of sophisticated matching methods and their associated analytic strategies.

Despite the utility of traditional case-control designs for association, statistical geneticists recently have focused on within-family tests of association and linkage disequilibrium. The general rationale underlying the development of these within-family methods is that case-control methods—even the highly sophisticated contemporary varieties—are insufficient to fully ensure matching between cases and controls. In other words, difficulties inherent in adumbrating all possible confounder variables impede the success of matching as a strategy for eliminating all potential confounds in inferring the relation between a candidate gene and a disease. The failure to completely control for potential confounders results in problematic inferences regarding the association between a gene and a disorder or trait being attributable to the *causal effects* of the gene, rather than to some concomitant variable. The most conspicuous confounding variables are sources of population stratification, such as ethnicity or SES, that induce correlations between a gene and a disorder that are due to allele frequencies and rates of disorders differing across ethnic groups or SES levels, rather than to linkage.

Within-family tests of linkage and association avoid confounding caused by population stratification (Schaid and Sommer 1994; Spielman et al. 1993). It also is important to realize that any source of population stratification, not simply ethnic heterogeneity, may result in artifactual inferences regarding association (Ewens and Spielman 1995). An elegant and simple within-family association test, the transmission disequilibrium test (TDT), is based on the detection of unequal transmission of high- versus low-risk alleles by heterozygous parents to children with a specific behavioral trait or disorder. The Mendelian expectation under the null hypothesis is that either allele carried by a heterozygote has a 50:50 chance of transmission to that child. If the allele actually plays a role in the development of the behavioral trait or disorder, however, then its transmission should exceed 50 percent.

The TDT has certain advantages over other within-family association tests, e.g., affected family-based controls (Thomson 1995) and haplotype-based haplotype relative risk (HHRR) (Falk and Rubinstein 1987; Terwilliger and Ott 1992). These include (1) greater statistical power, (2) robustness against artifacts induced by population stratification, (3) a test of linkage in the presence of association, and (4) for the test of linkage (but not association), the ability to include multiple affected siblings from a family without having to correct for nonindependence (Schaid and Sommer 1994; Spielman et al. 1993). Given these features, researchers have begun to rely on within-family analyses using the TDT as a primary source of evidence regarding association and linkage between candidate genes and disorders.

Because of the statistical properties of the TDT, it can easily be extended to examine moderators of association and linkage. Such extensions have been developed using log-linear analysis for the case of categorical moderators, such as sex or diagnostic subtype (Waldman et al. 1997b), and logistic regression for the case of moderation by continuous variables, such as symptom severity, age of onset, and symptoms of co-morbid disorders (Waldman et al. 1997a). Extensions of the TDT using the t-test (Allison 1997) and logistic regression (Waldman et al. 1997a) also have been developed for examining association and linkage of a candidate gene with a continuous variable.

Of the three methods described, linkage analysis, allele-sharing studies, and association/linkage disequilibrium, the latter may be the most powerful and practical for identifying genes for behavioral traits or disorders. Using simulation studies, it has been shown that linkage and allele-sharing methods may only be useful when a locus has a substantial genetic effect ($\geq$ 10–15% of the liability variance) (Risch and Merikangas 1996; Suarez et al. 1994). In contrast, the TDT may be able to identify loci with a much smaller effect with a reasonable sample size. Moreover, this approach is less limiting regarding the types of families sampled because single affected offspring and their parents are informative. Extensions of this test to incorporate families without parents (e.g., siblings only) are under development and thus the TDT or similar tests could be applied to late-onset disorders.

Experimental Crosses in Animal Systems

It appears that most behavioral traits are influenced by many genes, each with a relatively weak effect. Detecting these genes may be difficult using most of the approaches outlined above, primarily because of their reduced power in the human system resulting from small families and genetic and environmental heterogeneity. The use of experimental model systems can circumvent these problems. One approach that takes advantage of such systems is quantitative trait locus (QTL) analysis (Lander and Botestein 1986). This approach is most effective in animals or plants for which there are inbred strains. For example, mice and rats are being used to identify genes that may be involved in anxiety (Flint et al. 1995).

The basic approach is to mate two inbred lines that differ in some trait (e.g., anxiety), to generate the first generation (F_1) of hybrid animals. The resulting hybrid animal has one set of genes from the serene parent and one from the anxious parent. The F_1 animals are then mated back to the parental inbred strain of serene animals, resulting in F_2 offspring with one recombinant set of chromosomes and one pure set from the serene inbred strain. The recombinant chromosome set is unique for each F_2 offspring owing to the recombination that occurs in a random fashion along each chromosome arm. Because each offspring carries a different portion of the genome from the anxious mouse strain, they will vary with respect to anxiety. To detect putative genes, a random set of genetic markers with alleles that differ between the two strains along each chromosome are genotyped. At each marker, animals are separated into two groups: (1) those with an allele from the anxious strain and (2) those with an allele from the serene strain. Scores for anxiety in those two groups are then compared. If there is a difference between the two groups in the phenotype, that chromosome region is a candidate region for a gene that influences anxious behavior. The search then continues for other such markers. As with the methods described previously, choosing a critical value to indicate significance is difficult because of the unknown underlying genetic structure and the large number of tests conducted (see later discussion).

Another approach involving model systems is mentioned here although it is not used to detect a putative gene, but to determine if a behavioral phenotype results when a particular gene is inactivated or "knocked out." A powerful approach is to combine knockout animals with QTL analysis to identify modifying genes. Approaches using model systems should be thought of as tools to be used in concert with human studies, although they may or may not be representative of the human system. Nevertheless, findings from model systems can pinpoint important neurogenetic causal pathways that may be involved in specific behavioral phenotypes.

Strategies to Increase the Chance of Finding a Trait Gene

There are basically two general strategies for finding genes that influence a disorder or behavioral trait: (1) a brute-force, genome-wide scan, or (2) a study of candidate genes. The former involves genotyping an ordered set of markers spread equidistantly throughout the genome. The latter examines polymorphisms in specific genes that potentially are involved in the etiology of the trait or disorder. There are advocates of both approaches and researchers who do a little of both.

The obvious advantage of a genome-wide scan is that eventually previously unknown loci will be identified and putative genes isolated; that is, a large net is cast to find a susceptibility gene. Genome-wide scans are enormous undertakings, however. The size of the task depends on the magnitude of the gene's effect, the statistical approach taken, and the type of population examined (see later discussion). Alternatively, in a candidate gene approach, only genes hypothesized to play a role in the etiology of the trait are tested for linkage or associations. Given the definition of a candidate gene, only tight linkage (i.e., $\theta \approx$ 0) is tested. The loss of power that often results in a genome-wide scan using markers spaced 20 centimorgans (cM) apart does not occur in a candidate gene approach. More important, if evidence for a candidate gene is found, a tremendous amount of knowledge is gained, because the function of the gene is already known. Obviously, this approach is being applied more often as the number of genes with known functions increases.

The structure of the population plays an important role in linkage studies. Various designs can be considered, depending on the analytical approach chosen. For studies using linkage analyses, a single large family or families from genetically isolated populations has the advantage of reducing genetic heterogeneity, but also has the possible disadvantage of limited representation of the general population. For genome-wide scans, statistical power increases if "young" populations with recent founders are studied, because linkage disequilibrium remains over larger chromosomal distances flanking a putative gene (Houwen et al. 1994). Thus, the typical reduction in power caused by the genetic distance between the marker and the trait gene is minimized. Of course, the ease of collecting from only affected individuals and their parents (i.e., for the TDT), versus affected relatives (i.e., for APM), versus full extended families (i.e., for traditional linkage studies) must be taken into account, given the behavioral trait or disorder to be studied.

Statistical Significance

Lander and Kruglyak (1995, 241) lay out the methodological problem of identifying a putative gene for a complex trait. As they describe it, detection of a putative gene involved in a simple or complex trait "boils down to finding those chromosome regions that tend to be shared among affected relatives and tend to differ between affecteds and unaffecteds. Conceptually, this amounts to a three-step recipe: scan the entire genome with a dense collection of genetic markers; calculate an appropriate linkage statistic $S(x)$ at each position x along the genome; and identify the regions in which the statistic S shows a significant deviation from what would be expected under independent assortment." Although their recipe may be simple, the choice of a critical value to declare a significant deviation from the null hypothesis is complicated, especially in genome-wide scans. For complex disorders, this issue remains largely unresolved. The traditional thresholds of a lod score of 3 for model-based linkage analyses and a p-value of 0.001 for nonparametric-based methods are still used as guidelines. Examples can be given of linkage findings for psychiatric disorders that exceeded such thresholds (e.g., Egeland et al. 1987; Sherrington et al. 1988) but failed to replicate. Because the underlying genetic structure of most behavioral traits is not known, there is no theoretical basis for establishing a critical value for significance, especially for genomic scans.

Lander and Kruglyak (1995) offer guidelines with justifications and also limitations to their use. They state that for genome-wide scans there is a 5 percent chance of randomly finding a region with a p-value as extreme as 2×10^{-5}. Therefore, to keep the chance of detecting a false positive at no more than 5 percent, critical values of Z score ≥ 4.1, lod score ≥ 3.6 or $p \leq 2 \times 10^{-5}$ should be used. In the past, standards for reporting results based on the significance levels were developed and maintained by the genetics community and were reiterated by Lander and Kruglyak. That is, there should be different levels of confidence for the linkage between a putative disease gene and genetic marker, depending on the statistical significance of the finding. Suggestive, significant, and highly significant levels would relate to statistical evidence that would be expected to occur 1, 0.05, and 0.001 times at random in a genome scan, respectively. Confirmed linkage would only be declared if an initial significant linkage was replicated in an independent sample at a level of $p \leq 0.01$. The critical value can be reduced in confirmation studies because usually the studies are based on testing a single chromosomal region, rather than multiple regions.

Failure to replicate a linkage finding does not necessarily mean that the initial finding is a false positive. For weak gene effects (e.g., 10%), Suarez et al. (1994) show that the first positive linkage results are somewhat biased. They include the effects of chance to help push the evidence over the critical value. Subsequent studies will not contain this bias and will regress to the true value.

For that reason, it takes a much larger sample to replicate an initial finding. Reporting the power of the sample to detect linkage would help evaluate negative results. There are other factors that complicate replicating positive findings, including population heterogeneity, diagnostic differences, and methodology (e.g., specification of genetic models).

The theoretical p-values just described are based on large-sample, asymptotic theory. If the sample is not large enough or if other assumptions of the statistic do not hold, the theoretical p-value may not be correct. To avoid this problem, another approach to evaluating statistical significance has been suggested. This consists of using computer simulation to generate an empirical distribution of the statistic under the null hypothesis of no linkage based on the trait phenotype and pedigree structure of the family data set (e.g., Schroeder et al. 1996). For example, for genetic linkage studies, each set of simulated data is generated by simulating an unlinked marker that is transmitted through each family in the data set. The lod score is then estimated using the original trait phenotype and the simulated marker genotypes. This simulation is done many times to generate the empirical distribution, and the p-value for the observed test statistic is taken from the empirical distribution. Such resampling methods yield a test statistic that is much less dependent on the usual assumptions underlying parametric statistics.

Recent Findings of Genes Involved in Behavioral Traits or Disorders

There are many examples in the literature that illustrate both successes and failures in detecting genes involved in psychiatric disorders or behavioral traits. A similar record can be found for any complex trait, although the news media coverage for behavioral traits seems to be more sensationalized. Even judicious restraint in the interpretation of positive results by some authors can be undermined by the lay press or the scientific community. In the next sections we present a few important examples of such findings, the approaches used, the results, and the interpretations of those results.

Schizophrenia: Linkage Analysis as the Primary Approach

In 1995, linkage of a marker on chromosome 6 to one of the possible susceptibility genes involved in the etiology of schizophrenia was reported (Straub et al. 1995). Two reports replicated the finding (Moises et al. 1995;

Schwab et al. 1995) and three did not (Antonarakis et al. 1995; Gurling et al. 1995; Mowry et al. 1995). These reports came after earlier failures to replicate a reported linkage on chromosome 5 (Sherrington et al. 1988), so it is not surprising that the chromosome 6 findings were greeted with some skepticism.

In the majority of studies on schizophrenia, linkage analysis has been used as the primary tool to identify susceptibility genes, although the underlying genetic structure of schizophrenia is not known. Recently, researchers have used a variety of analytical methods to support their linkage findings. The strategy used in the leading paper of the recent series mentioned earlier (Straub et al. 1995) exemplifies the idea of assessing the support for linkage under various genetic models and methodological approaches, and seeking replication by other investigators. The authors used careful psychiatric diagnostic criteria based on standardized techniques. The effect of the definition of an affected individual on the support for linkage was investigated using a hierarchical approach, in that analyses were conducted assuming a narrow, intermediate, or broad definition of schizophrenia and, finally, an all-inclusive definition (i.e., all psychiatric disorders).

Similar to almost all linkage studies of schizophrenia to date, Straub et al. modeled the underlying genetic component for schizophrenia as a single gene that accounted for the greater part of genetic variance. Multiple genes, epistasis, environmental factors, and gene-environment interactions were not included. They examined the support for linkage under several single gene models, including dominant, co-dominant, additive liability, and recessive models (see the table in the Methods section in Straub et al. 1995). Parameters to define such models were fixed, whereas the admixture parameter, or the proportion of pedigrees segregating the disease locus, was estimated with the recombination fraction. The highest lod score, assuming genetic heterogeneity, of 3.51 was found with D6S296.

The positive findings from the initial linkage analysis were followed by an affecteds-only analysis to determine the influence of unaffected individuals in the families. Next, a C-test (Maclean et al. 1992) was performed. This analysis is based on the sum of individual pedigree maximum lod scores combined with a bootstrap method of estimating the null hypothesis distribution (i.e., for the model assuming no linkage). These model-based analyses were followed by a nonparametric approach using an extended sibling pair analysis.

The criterion used for significance was carefully considered. Although a total of 320 tests were performed, no correction for multiple testing was done because it was noted that such tests were not independent, and common corrections (e.g., Bonferroni correction) would be too conservative. The authors stated that the highest lod score obtained, 3.5, would be followed up in the same manner, irrespective of some correction factor: that is, prior to publication, the authors communicated the detailed results of their findings to others in the field to facilitate replication studies.

One of the studies that was able to replicate the positive findings of linkage on chromosome 6 was by Moises et al. (1995). They used a two-stage approach to detect linkage, one that is becoming widely used. In general, in the first stage the genome is scanned with markers that are relatively far apart (e.g., 20 cM) to identify suggestive linkage. In the second stage those suggestive linkages are followed up with more densely mapped markers in the candidate regions identified. In the study by Moises et al. (1995), a model-free linkage analysis of large pedigrees was used in their first stage of the study, and 26 loci that were suggestive of linkage ($p \leq 0.05$) were found. In the second stage, 10 of the 26 chromosome regions with the lowest p-values and/or those with flanking loci suggesting linkage were followed up in a second independent data set. Four of these 10 markers again showed evidence for linkage. However, none reached the most stringent level of significance for linkage ($p \leq 0.0001$). A third sample was evaluated using fine mapping of 13 markers flanking the chromosome 6 region by association studies. Significant findings for the association test were found in this sample ($p \leq 0.05$), and combination of this sample with others from the literature produced significance ($p \leq 0.00004$).

To summarize, linkage analysis was successfully used to identify a putative susceptibility gene for schizophrenia, in spite of the problems associated with the lack of knowledge regarding the underlying genetic structure. However, other model-free approaches were used together with linkage analysis to fortify the conclusions, as in the careful study by Straub et al. (1995). Thus, linkage analysis may continue to play a role in identifying putative behavioral genes but perhaps only when it is used with other methods less sensitive to specified models.

Success of Allele-Sharing Methods in Identifying Susceptibility Genes for Reading Disability

Reading disability, or dyslexia, is a significant social, educational, and mental health problem that can profoundly affect children and adults with otherwise normal cognitive skills. One estimate of the number of children classified as reading disabled by the school system criteria is 8 percent (Rumsey 1992; Shaywitz et al. 1990). Many family and twin studies consistently have shown that genetic factors play a role in the etiology of this condition, although the exact mechanism(s) has not been delineated. It is clear that reading disability is a complex, etiologically heterogeneous disorder. Variability in the definition of the trait complicates studies of genetic as well as environmental influences.

The first study that attempted to locate genes involved in the etiology of reading disabilities was conducted in 1983 (Smith et al. 1983). The authors conducted a linkage analysis of nine three-generation families selected because of a family history of reading disabilities. An individual was defined as reading disabled if his or her reading level was at least two years below his or her expected grade level and he or she had an IQ greater than 90. The trait was modeled as a single-gene, dominant disorder. A genome-wide scan was performed using the limited number of polymorphic markers and chromosome heteromorphisms available at that time. A significant lod score ($Z = 3.24$ at $\theta = 0.13$) was found with a chromosome 15 heteromorphism. The authors were cautious in interpreting their finding as an identified genetic component for reading disability because of the complexity of the phenotype. Since that initial report, several studies have been undertaken to identify susceptibility genes. However, further linkage analyses of an augmented sample studied by Smith et al. (1983) and other samples failed to show linkage to chromosome 15 (Rabin et al. 1993; Smith and Kimberling 1991).

The original team of investigators followed up an interesting association of dyslexia and autoimmune disorders and, using a candidate gene approach, found a suggestion of linkage to the HLA complex on chromosome 6 (Rabin et al. 1993; Smith and Kimberling 1991). For a subsequent study, they targeted this candidate region using their augmented set of 19 families that segregated for the reading phenotype in an autosomal dominant pattern, as well as a twin sample drawn from 50 families (Cardon et al. 1994). A continuous measure of reading performance that was based on discriminant function weights for reading recognition, reading comprehension, and spelling was used as a more precise phenotype. A nonparametric sibling pair approach that was extended to accommodate interval mapping (i.e., examining a genetic interval bounded by two genetic markers instead of examining one marker at a time) was performed. The authors also used two extensions of the DeFries and Fulker regression model to replace the conventional sibling-pair analysis. Although the details of this method are beyond the scope of this chapter, in general the method involves regressing the score for one sibling onto (1) the score for the second sibling, (2) the proportion of alleles that the sibling pairs share identical by descent at the marker locus, and (3) the product of those two variables. The different statistical approaches on the two independent samples of sibling pairs provided evidence for a quantitative trait locus on chromosome 6 within a 2-cM region of the HLA complex. The combined evidence from both samples was significant at $p = 0.0002$.

This work was followed by a study that was able to replicate the chromosome 6 linkage and to suggest an additional linkage on chromosome 15 (Grigorenko et al. 1997). These authors used both parametric (linkage analysis) and nonparametric (APM) methods and extended the investigation by dissecting the phenotype of reading disability into five theoretically derived phenotypes: (1) phonological awareness, (2) phonological decoding, (3) rapid automatized naming, (4) single-word reading, and (5) discrepancy between intelligence and reading performance. They found significant evidence ($p \leq 10^{-6}$) for linkage between the phonological awareness phenotype and chromosome 6 markers, whereas the phenotype defined as single-word reading provided the least compelling evidence for linkage of all five traits. In contrast, suggestive linkage ($Z = 3.15$, $\theta = 0.0$) between single-word reading and a chromosome 15 marker was identified, whereas the analyses with the phonological awareness phenotype were negative.

Thus, as shown with schizophrenia, the use of several approaches to detect putative behavioral genes is essential. For detecting genes for reading disabilities, methods based on allele-sharing were used, some of which were extended in innovative ways. Moreover, the study by Grigorenko et al. (1997) examined the components of the behavioral trait and was able to show that linkage appeared to be at least somewhat specific for different components of reading disability.

QTL Analysis in Experimental Animals Uncovers
Putative Genes for Anxiety

As demonstrated with reading disability, the phenotypes of many traits can be dissected into their component parts. Some psychological traits are defined by the covariation of a set of behavioral measures that otherwise appear to have little in common. Emotionality in mice is an example of such a trait. Flint et al. (1995) defined emotionality as the covariation of open-field activity (OFA) and defecation in a novel environment and emergence into the open arms of an elevated plus maze. They conducted a large QTL analysis of these anxiety measures. One goal of this study was to examine the hypothesis that these behaviors in mice are analogous to anxiety in humans by finding QTLs that were related to the set of behaviors and explain the correlations among them.

The experiment had two stages. First, Flint et al. (1995) conducted a QTL study using inbred mouse strains derived from animals selected for both high and low defecation with OFA, a phenotype related to emotionality in mice. In the second stage, they determined if the putative genes for OFA could explain the other correlated measures that together defined emotionality. Briefly, they found that a small number of loci with relatively large effects appear to explain a large portion (25%) of the genetic variance of OFA in the mouse. In addition, some of these genes seemed to explain the genetic variance of the correlated measures used to define emotionality. Thus, the same QTLs appeared to influence four different behavioral measures. The authors were able to define the location within the mouse genome of three of these loci that contributed substantially to the genetic variance of emotionality. Now the challenge is to define the nature of these genes and then to determine if emotionality in mice is representative of the psychological trait of anxiety in humans.

Uses of Within-Family Tests of Linkage Disequilibrium and Association

Analyses of association and linkage disequilibrium have yielded positive findings in a number of areas of both medical and psychiatric genetics. Although some of these methods (e.g., traditional case-control comparisons) have the disadvantage of susceptibility to potential confounds, both population and within-family association methods often can be more powerful than traditional linkage analyses. For example, although linkage analyses of Alzheimer disease yielded findings that were only marginal for the ApoE allele, population association methods produced strong findings (Strittmatter et al. 1993).

Within-family tests of linkage disequilibrium also have yielded important findings for a number of medical diseases and psychiatric disorders. An example of a medical disease in which such methods were instrumental is the relation between insulin-dependent diabetes mellitus (IDDM) and the insulin gene region on chromosome 11p. Similar to the aforementioned case of Alzheimer disease and the ApoE allele, conventional linkage methods (e.g., co-segregation in affected sibling pairs) yielded findings that were weak, at times not even departing from random allele sharing, despite evidence of a population association (Cox and Spielman 1989). In contrast, within-family tests of linkage disequilibrium using the TDT provided strong evidence for linkage and association between IDDM and a polymorphism adjacent to the insulin gene region (Spielman et al. 1993).

In the domain of psychiatric disorders, within-family tests of association and linkage disequilibrium recently have played an important role in suggesting a relation between childhood attention deficit hyperactivity disorder (ADHD) and the dopamine transporter gene (DAT1). This is a good candidate gene for ADHD because its product, dopamine transporter, regulates the amount of dopamine active in a synapse and is a primary target of psychostimulant medications such as Ritalin, which are among the most effective treatments for ADHD. Further evidence suggesting the importance of DAT1 for ADHD comes from a "knockout gene" study in mice (Giros et al. 1996). In this study, mice who were homozygous for deactivation of the DAT1 allele were 5 to 6 times more active and had dopamine remain active in the synaptic cleft 100 times longer than heterozygous and wild-type mice.

Association of the dopamine transporter gene and ADHD was initially reported using HHRR (Cook et al. 1995) and then extended to linkage disequilibrium using the TDT on data from the same sample (Cook et al. 1997). Although this association was not replicated in a subsequent study using a relatively small, less severely affected sample (LaHoste et al. 1995), a recent replication of association using HHRR has been reported (Gill et al. 1997).

In addition, Waldman et al. (1997a) replicated and extended the finding of linkage disequilibrium between ADHD and DAT1. Evidence for association and linkage between ADHD and DAT1 was found using between-family and within-family analyses. Specifically, the number of DAT1 high-risk alleles was linearly related to both the inattentive and hyperactive-impulsive symptoms of ADHD, and siblings who were genetically discordant for the number of DAT1 high-risk alleles differed dramatically in their scores on scales for each of these symptom dimensions. Based on evidence from TDT tests, DAT1 was significantly related to the combined subtype of ADHD, which requires surpassing symptom thresholds on both the inattentive and hyperactive-impulsive symptom dimensions, but not to the inattentive subtype of ADHD, which requires surpassing the symptom threshold on the inattentive but not the hyperactive-impulsive symptom dimension. This suggests that DAT1 may have some specificity to the hyperactive-impulsive symptoms of ADHD and highlights the importance of defining specific phenotypes in psychiatric molecular genetic studies, which is similar to recent findings for reading disability (Grigorenko et al. 1997).

In another example, an association of the serotonin transporter gene (5HTT) and anxiety-related personality traits (e.g., neuroticism) was reported using both between- and within-family analyses (Lesch et al. 1996). This is a good candidate gene for anxiety-related traits because transporter-mediated reuptake of serotonin has been suggested and found to affect anxiety levels in both humans and animals (Lesch et al. 1996). In addition, a number of recently developed antianxiety and antidepressant medications have serotonin reuptake as a primary target of action. In between-family analyses, Lesch et al. (1996) found that individuals with one or two copies of the 5HTT short allele had higher scores on the anxiety-related personality traits (e.g., anxiety, angry hostility, depression, impulsiveness, tension, and suspiciousness) than individuals with two copies of the long allele. The authors followed up these analyses with within-family analyses of genetically discordant sibling pairs, and found that siblings with one or two copies of the 5HTT short allele had significantly higher scores on neuroticism, tension, and harm avoidance than their cosiblings with two long alleles. These findings are interesting given the results in mice by Flint et al. (1995), who found a number of QTLs that influence levels of emotionality.

Summary

With current and anticipated genetic resources, technological advances, and statistical developments, genes that influence the susceptibility of complex traits will be detected. They are genes that do not act on their own, but interact with one or many genes and environmental factors. On their own, they explain only a small portion of the variance of the complex phenotype. Behavioral traits and disorders clearly fall into the category of complex traits from this genetic viewpoint. In this chapter, we have highlighted the implications of genetic complex traits in terms of research design and analysis and provided a few examples of successful investigations that have applied these techniques to behavioral traits and psychiatric disorders. The statistical complexities of such analyses were noted. One exciting development has been the addition of new statistical methods (e.g., TDT and its extensions) to the armament of more traditional methods of linkage analysis and allele sharing. In the near future, these new methods will work hand-in-hand with technological advances in the automation of genotyping (e.g., DNA "chip" technology) and allow massive genome searches with relatively little effort. The continued challenge will be to refine or dissect the phenotypes of behavioral traits and psychiatric disorders to facilitate the identification of putative genes and to uncover their complicated interactions with the environment. Ultimately, we may begin to understand the basis of the neurological pathways leading to human behaviors.

References

Allison, D. B. 1997. Transmission-disequilibrium tests for quantitative traits. *Am. J. Hum. Genet.* 60: 676–690.

Amos, C. I., D. V. Dawson, and R. C. Elston. 1990. The probabilistic determination of identity-by-descent sharing for pairs of relatives from pedigrees. *Am. J. Hum. Genet.* 47: 842–853.

Amos, C. I., D. K. Zhu, and E. Boerwinkle. 1996. Assessing genetic linkage and association with robust components of variance approaches. *Ann. Hum. Genet.* 60: 143–160.

Antonarakis, S. E., J. L. Blouin, A. E. Pulver, et al. 1995. Schizophrenia susceptibility and chromosome 6p24–22. *Nat. Genet.* 11: 235–236.

Baron, M., N. Risch, R. Hamburger, et al. 1987. Genetic linkage between X-chromosome markers and bipolar affective illness. *Nature* 326: 289–292.

Baron, M., N. R. Freimer, N. Risch, et al. 1993. Diminished support for linkage between manic depressive illness and X-chromosome markers in three Israeli pedigrees. *Nat. Genet.* 3: 49–55.

Bonney, G. E. 1986. Regressive logistic models for familial disease and other binary traits. *Biometry* 42: 611–625.

Brunner, H. G., M. R. Nelen, P. van Zandvort, et al. 1993. X-linked borderline mental retardation with prominent behavioral disturbance: Phenotype, genetic localization, and evidence for disturbed monoamine metabolism. *Am. J. Hum. Genet.* 52: 1032–1039.

Cardon, L. R., S. D. Smith, D. W. Fulker, et al. 1994. Quantitative trait locus for reading disability on chromosome 6. *Science* 266: 276–279.

Cook, E. H., Jr., M. A. Stein, M. D. Krasowski, et al. 1995. Association of attention-deficit disorder and the dopamine transporter gene. *Am. J. Hum. Genet.* 56: 993–998.

Cook, E. H., Jr., M. A. Stein, and B. L. Leventhal. 1997. Family-based association of attention-deficit/hyperactivity disorder and the dopamine transporter. In *Handbook of Psychiatric Genetics*, K. Blum and E. Noble, eds. Boca Raton, Fla.: CRC Press.

Cox, N. J., and R. S. Spielman. 1989. The insulin gene and susceptibility of IDDM. *Genet. Epidemiol.* 6: 65–89.

DeFries, J. C., and D. W. Fulker. 1985. Multiple regression analysis of twin data. *Behav. Genetics* 15: 467–473.

DeFries, J. C., and D. W. Fulker. 1988. Multiple regression analysis of twin data: Etiology of deviant scores versus individual differences. *Acta Genet. Med. Gemellol.* 37: 205–216.

Egeland, J. A., D. S. Gerhard, D. L. Pauls, et al. 1987. Bipolar affective disorders linked to DNA markers on chromosome 11. *Nature* 325: 783–787.

Ewens, W. J., and R. S. Spielman. 1995. The transmission/disequilibrium test: History, subdivision, and admixture. *Am. J. Hum. Genet.* 57: 455–464.

Falk, C. T., and P. Rubinstein. 1987. Haplotype relative risks: An easy reliable way to construct a proper control sample for risk calculations. *Ann. Hum. Genet.* 51: 227–233.

Flint, J., R. Corley, J. C. DeFries, et al. 1995. A simple genetic basis for a complex psychological trait in laboratory mice. *Science* 269: 1432–1435.

Gill, M., G. Daly, S. Heron, et al. 1997. Confirmation of association between attention deficit hyperactivity disorder and a dopamine transporter polymorphism. *Mol. Psychiatry* 2: 311–313.

Giros, B., M. Jaber, S. R. Jones, et al. 1996. Hyperlocomotion and indifference to cocaine and amphetamine in mice lacking the dopamine transporter. *Nature* 379: 606–612.

Grigorenko, E. L., F. B. Wood, M. S. Meyer, et al. 1997. Susceptibility loci for distinct components of developmental dyslexia on chromosomes 6 and 15. *Am. J. Hum. Genet.* 60: 27–39.

Gurling, H., G. Kalsi, A. Hui-Sui Chen, et al. 1995. Schizophrenia susceptibility and chromosome 6p24–22. *Nat. Genet.* 11: 234–235.

Haseman, J. K., and R. C. Elston. 1972. The investigation of linkage between a quantitative trait and marker locus. *Behav. Genet.* 2: 3–19.

Houwen, R. H., S. Baharloo, K. Blankenship, et al. 1994. Genome screening by searching for shared segments: Mapping a gene for benign recurrent intrahepatic cholestasis. *Nature Genet.* 8: 380–386.

Kelsoe, J. R., E. I. Ginns, J. A. Egeland, et al. 1989. Re-evaluation of the linkage relationship between chromosome 11p loci and the gene for bipolar affective disorder in the Old Order Amish. *Nature* 342: 238–243.

Kennedy, J. L. 1988. Evidence against linkage of schizophrenia to markers on chromosome 5 in a northern Swedish pedigree. *Nature* 336: 167–170.

Kruglyak, L., and E. S. Lander. 1995. Complete multipoint sib-pair analysis of quali-tative and quantitative traits. *Am. J. Hum. Genet.* 57: 439–454.

LaHoste, G. J., S. B. Wigal, C. Glabe, et al. 1995. Dopamine-related genes and atten-tion deficit hyperactivity disorder. Paper presented at the annual meeting of the Society for the Neurosciences, San Diego. 1995 (Abstract).

Lander, E. S., and D. Botestein. 1986. Mapping complex genetic traits in humans: New methods using a complete RFLP linkage map. *Cold Spring Harbor Symposia on Quantitative Biology,* 49. Cold Spring Harbor Laboratory, N.Y.: Cold Spring Harbor Press.

Lander, E. S., and N. J. Schork. 1994. Genetic dissection of complex traits. *Science* 265: 2037–2048.

Lander, E., and L. Kruglyak. 1995. Genetic dissection of complex traits: Guidelines for interrupting and reporting linkage results. *Nat. Genet.* 11: 241–247.

Lesch, K. P., D. Bengel, A. Heils, et al. 1996. Association of anxiety-related traits with a polymorphism in the serotonin transporter gene regulatory region. *Science* 274: 1527–1531.

Maclean, C. J., L. M. Ploughman, S. R. Diehl, et al. 1992. A new test for linkage in the presence of locus heterogeneity. *Am. J. Hum. Genet.* 50: 1259–1266.

Moises, H. W., L. Yang, H. Kristbjarnarson, et al. 1995. An international two-stage genome-wide search for schizophrenia susceptibility genes. *Nat. Genet.* 11: 321–324.

Mowry, B. J., D. J. Nancarrow, D. P. Lennon, et al. 1995. Schizophrenia susceptibility and chromosome 6p24–22. *Nat. Genet.* 11: 233–236.

Neale, M. C., and L. R. Cardon. 1992. *Methodology for Genetic Studies of Twins and Families.* Boston: Kluwer Academic.

Pericak-Vance, M. A., J. L. Bebout, P. C. J. Gaskell, et al. 1991. Linkage studies in fa-milial Alzheimer's disease: Evidence for chromosome 19 linkage. *Am. J. Hum. Genet.* 48: 1034–1050.

Rabin, M., X. L. Wen, M. Hepburn, et al. 1993. Suggestive linkage of developmental dyslexia to chromosome 1p34–p36. *Lancet* 342: 178.

Risch, N., and K. Merikangas. 1996. The future of genetic studies of complex human diseases. *Science* 273: 1516–1517.

Risch, N., and H. Zhang. 1995. Extreme discordant sib pairs for mapping quantita-tive trait loci in humans. *Science* 268: 1584–1589.

Rumsey, J. M. 1992. The biology of developmental dyslexia. *J. Am. Med. Assoc.* 19: 912–915.

Schaid, D. J., and S. S. Sommer. 1994. Comparison of statistics for candidate-gene as-sociation studies using cases and parents. *Am. J. Hum. Genet.* 55: 402–409.

Schroeder, D. S., L. R. Goldin, and D. E. Weeks. 1996. Nonparametric simulation-based statistics for detecting linkage in general pedigrees. *Am. J. Hum. Genet.* 58: 867–880.

Schwab, S. G., M. Albus, J. Hallmayer, et al. 1995. Evaluation of a susceptibility gene for schizophrenia on chromosome 6p by multipoint affected sib-pair linkage analysis. *Nat. Genet.* 11: 325–327.

Shaywitz, S. E., B. A. Shaywitz, J. M. Fletcher, and M. D. Escobar. 1990. Prevalence of reading disability in boys and girls. *J. Am. Med. Assoc.* 264: 998–1002.

Sherrington, R., J. Brynjolfsson, H. Petursson, et al. 1988. Localization of a susceptibility locus for schizophrenia on chromosome 5. *Nature* 336: 164–170.

Smith, S. D., and W. J. Kimberling. 1991. *Reading Disabilities: Genetic and Neurobiological Influences.* Boston: Kluwer Academic.

Smith, S. D., W. J. Kimberling, B. F. Pennington, and H. A. Lubs. 1983. Specific reading disability: Identification of an inherited form through linkage analysis. *Science* 219: 1345–1347.

Spielman, R. S., R. E. McGinnis, and W. J. Ewens. 1993. Transmission test for linkage disequilibrium: The insulin gene region and insulin-dependent diabetes mellitus (IDDM). *Am. J. Hum. Genet.* 52: 506–516.

Straub, R. E., C. J. Maclean, F. A. O'Neill, et al. 1995. A potential vulnerability locus for schizophrenia on chromosome 6p24–22: Evidence for genetic heterogeneity. *Nat. Genet.* 11: 287–293.

Strittmatter, W. J., A. M. Saunders, D. Schmechel, et al. 1993. Apolipoprotein E: High-avidity binding to b-amyloid and increased frequency of type 4 allele in late-onset familial Alzheimer disease. *Proc. Natl. Acad. Sci. U.S.A.* 90: 1977–1981.

Suarez, B. K., C. L. Hampe, and P. VanEerdewegh. 1994. Problems of replicating linkage claims in psychiatry. In *Genetic Approaches to Mental Disorders*, E. S. Gershon and C. R. Cloninger, eds., 23. Washington, D.C.: American Psychiatric Association.

Terwilliger, J. D., and J. Ott. 1992. A haplotype-based "haplotype relative risk" approach to detecting allelic associations. *Hum. Hered.* 42: 337–346.

Thomson, G. 1995. Mapping disease genes: Family-based association studies. *Am. J. Hum. Genet.* 57: 487–498.

Verkerk, A. J., M. Pieretti, J. S. Sutcliffe, et al. 1991. Identification of a gene (FMR-1) containing a CGG repeat coincident with a breakpoint cluster region exhibiting length variation in fragile X syndrome. *Cell* 65: 905–914.

Waldman, I. D., B. F. Robinson, and S. A. Feigon. 1997a. Linkage disequilibrium between the dopamine transporter gene (DAT1) and bipolar disorder: Extending the transmission disequilibrium test (TDT) to examine genetic heterogeneity. *Genet. Epidemiol.* 14: 699–704.

Waldman, I. D., M. B. Miller, B. F. Robinson, et al. 1997b. A continuous variable TDT using logistic regression analysis. Paper presented at the annual meeting of the Behavior Genetics Association, Toronto, Ontario, Canada (Abstract).

Wang, S., C. Sun, C. A. Walczak, et al. 1995. Evidence for a susceptibility locus for schizophrenia on chromosome 6pter-p22. *Nat. Genet.* 10: 41–46.

Weeks, D. E., and K. Lange. 1988. The affected-pedigree-member method of linkage analysis. *Am. J. Hum. Genet.* 42: 315–326.

Weeks, D. E., and G. M. Lathrop. 1995. Polygenic disease: Methods for mapping complex traits. *Trends Genet.* 11: 513–519.

4 Complexity and Research Strategies in Behavioral Genetics

Kenneth F. Schaffner, M.D., Ph.D.

Behavioral genetics has advanced rapidly in recent years (Kelner and Benditt 1994), and psychiatric genetics, in spite of some setbacks in the 1980s, is actively pursuing a behavioral genetic research program (Bock and Goode 1996; Gershon and Cloninger 1994). However, these advances and ongoing research projects are both problematic and contentious to many individuals and to some groups. As Nobel Laureate Thorsten Wiesel wrote, "Perhaps most disturbing to our sense of being free individuals, capable to a large degree of shaping our character and our minds, is the idea that our behavior, mental abilities, and mental health can be determined or destroyed by a segment of DNA" (Wiesel 1994, 1647). The appearance of Herrnstein and Murray's *The Bell Curve* in late 1994 and the reaction to it (some of the printed reaction is gathered in two anthologies: Fraser 1995 and Jacoby and Glauberman 1995) represent one facet of this contentiousness. *The Bell Curve* also drew a response from the National Institute of Health's Working Group (Andrews and Nelkin 1996). Another highly fractious example revolved around the University of Maryland's project on genetics and criminal behavior, and especially the September 1995 conference. That conference was invaded by several dissident groups, who then had to be escorted off the conference premises by the authorities (Editorial 1995).

This chapter does not dwell on these more contentious examples, because I believe that they do not represent the best of behavioral and psychiatric genetics. Much of the research underlying *The Bell Curve* and studies of criminality and antisocial behavior is based on an earlier paradigm of behavioral genetics: twin, relative, and adoption studies that may confound genetics and environment by relying on a questionable "heritability" concept.[1] The approach here, rather, is to try to provide a philosophical framework within which to interpret some of the most recent and exciting advances in behavioral and psychiatric genetics that use a molecular point of view.

This chapter, however, is not a paean to a reductionism, and in particular not to a *genetic* reductionism. Rather, its themes point toward complexity, multilevel interactionism, and the critical role of environment and learning in explanations of and interventions in mental disorders. Part of what motivates an interest in genetics, particularly psychiatric genetics, is the hope that identification of the gene, or more likely genes, contributing to serious mental disorders may give us information that we can use to diagnose and treat these disorders. This is based on the premise that an understanding of the molecular origin of a disorder such as schizophrenia or manic-depressive illness can simplify and clarify our approaches to existing illnesses. I have some doubts that such simplifications and clarifications will occur, but offer some suggestions for where we might look to achieve these hoped-for advances.

Can There Be Purely Genetic Explanations?

Before turning to the specifics of the genetics of behavioral traits, it is useful to clarify some terminology about genetic explanations, and especially to ask whether there can be any purely genetic explanations. The simple answer to this question is a "no." Genetic explanations are in all interesting cases incomplete. Even when characterized in detail at the DNA level, genes do not, all by themselves, explain much. The genes have to be translated into phenotypes, and typically have to function in a specified environment. Furthermore, genes do not act in a solitary manner—they act in concert with other genes, often with many genes. Thus, a genetic explanation needs to demarcate its limitations in explaining a phenotype, including a behavioral phenotype. The explanation must be situated in a broader context that recognizes that there are missing elements, such as environmental factors, even if they are not specific. It is largely these types of limitations, and the ignoring of them, that fuel much of the debate about genetic reductionism and determinism, a debate that is the backdrop to many of the issues facing this project on culture and biology.

The incompleteness of genetic explanations should not be surprising; this is the general consensus in the field of behavioral genetics and behavioral neuroscience. For example, a 1991 review by Kupferman in Kandel, Schwartz, and Jessel's *Principles of Neural Science*—a book that is a sort of bible of neuroscience—begins by noting that behavior in all organisms is shaped by the interaction of genes and environment. While the relative importance of the two factors varies, even the most stereotyped behavior can be modified by the environment, and most plastic behavior, such as language, is influenced by innate factors (Kupferman 1991, 987).[2] Kupferman then focuses on *aspects* of behavior (my italics) that might be inherited, and on the processes of interaction between genes and environment that affect behaviors. Thus the point about the incompleteness of any exclusively genetic basis for the explanation of behavior is taken as a general premise in the scientific community. (There are more radical claims against the primacy of a genetic component developed by those who take a "developmentalist" perspective, such as Gottleib [1992], Gray [1992], Griffiths and Gray [1994], and Oyama [1985], among others, that are considered briefly later.[3])

Scientists examining inherited aspects of behavior are especially interested in what ethologists such as Lorenz and Tinbergen originally called *instinctive behaviors*. These are now termed *species-specific behaviors* since they are the inherited characteristics of a species (Kupferman, 1991, 989). Lorenz and Tinbergen introduced two theoretical concepts to describe such behaviors: the cause (or releaser) of the behavior, termed the *sign stimulus*, and the stereotypical response of the organism, called the *fixed-action* pattern, often abbreviated as FAP.[4] An FAP can be quite complex, and in simple organisms the firing of a single command neuron can trigger activity in over a thousand different neurons in different neuronal subsystems. Such command neurons have been found in the crayfish and in *Aplysia* (Kupferman 1991, 990–991). Frost and Katz (1996) reported finding a single neuron in the marine mollusk *Tritonia diomedea* that triggers a long-lasting motor program governing the organism's escape swim. The input to command neurons is from a type of sensory neuron that detects specific features. It should be emphasized that though these types of behaviors are highly stereotypical, environmental factors and learning history can modify them to some extent. Thus, not even FAPs are set in concrete, although they are strong explainers of behavior. However, what triggers behavior, even in these simple systems, are single neurons, not single genes—not even a few genes. The point is an important one.

In spite of these caveats about the force of genetic explanation, there may be a sense in which a strong or primarily genetic explanation of behavior is appropriate. This would be limited to a behavior present when a gene(s) is present and absent when the gene(s) is absent (in an otherwise identical individual, subject to the same learning protocols, history, and environment).[5] We can approximate this idealized (impossibly idealized!) case by focusing on one relevant difference, in the context of otherwise gross similarity, to replace these overly stringent identity and difference conditions. This is similar to the case of a Huntington disease gene being present in an affected person but absent in an individual not carrying that gene. Some behavioral geneticists seem to believe that as we learn more about the molecular details underlying behavior, this type of single-gene paradigm, or a close oligogenetic (=a "few" genes) cousin of it, will receive significant support. This seems to inform much of the psychiatric genetic literature.

Two Recent Discoveries in Psychiatric / Mental Genetics

Two recent discoveries in the genetics of mental phenomena, one from the genetics of schizophrenia and the other from a genetic discovery involving a personality trait known as "novelty seeking," illustrate the problems of a purely genetic approach to mental illnesses. The following sections discuss some of the methodological problems with the research in these areas and argue that the genetics of mental health are best understood through a study of behavioral genetics. A review of recent advances in this area suggests potential problems as well as possible future successes in explaining and treating mental disorders.

Schizophrenia

Schizophrenia is a major mental disorder that occurs in approximately one out of every hundred individuals, a startlingly high prevalence for such a serious illness. It has been known for many years that the disorder runs in families, and a number of family, twin, and adoption studies have indicated that genetic factors are an important component. The 1980s saw several purported advances in the genetics both of schizophrenia and manic-depressive disorder, notably the localization of the former disease to chromosome 5 and the latter disorder to chromosome 11. Unfortunately, those results could not be confirmed, and these (probably) false positives have fueled criticisms of the entire effort to seek any precise genetic contribution to mental disorders. These false positive reports, however, have also engendered a much more sophisticated and critical approach to the methodology of studying complex traits, of which mental disorders are paradigms.

The November 1995 issue of *Nature Genetics* published three papers and three letters, four of which provide some fairly sound evidence for a schizophrenia vulnerability or susceptibility locus on the short arm of chromosome 6. These studies followed an earlier investigation by Straub and Kendler and their colleagues (Straub et al. 1995) that informally reported that preliminary evidence for a susceptibility locus for schizophrenia had been found in a sample of Irish schizophrenic families. In the main article in *Nature Genetics*, Straub and Kendler's group reported on an enlarged sample using 265 pedigrees and stated that "with linkage analysis we find evidence for a vulnerability locus for schizophrenia in the region 6p24–22. The greatest lod score, assuming locus heterogeneity, is 3.51 ($P = 0.0002$) with D6S296" (Straub et al. 1995, 287). (A lod score is a measure of the evidence in favor of a specific location for a trait-causing gene in comparison with a null hypothesis postulating no linkage to a trait-causing gene in the region [Lander and Schork 1994, 2039]. It is reported as a logarithm to the base 10 of the likelihood ratio, with a score of 3 typically taken as significant, although there are subtleties about this that are not detailed here.[6])

A paper by Moises et al. (1995) reports on a three-stage genome-wide search for a schizophrenia locus. In their first stage, they investigated five family lines in Iceland and found 26 loci that were suggestive of linkage. Ten of these loci were then followed up in stage II of their inquiry using a larger international set of 65 families. This stage provided potential linkages to chromosomes 6p, 9, and 20. The combination of the families from these two stages, and the addition of a third sample of 113 schizophrenics and their unaffected parents from China, yielded significant linkage to chromosome 6p. A study by Schwab et al. (1995) on affected sib pairs in 43 German families and 11 Israeli families, with a total of 78 sib pairs, reported a maximum lod score of 2.2 (indicating suggestive evidence) for a schizophrenia linkage to a region in chromosome 6. However, as Schwab et al. (1995, 326) note in comparing their results with Straub's investigation, there are clear differences in the *patterns* observed (my emphasis). A report by Antonarakis et al. (1995) also found a maximum lod score of 1.17, indicating at best suggestive evidence for chromosome 6. Two other studies by Mowry et al. (1995) and Gurling et al. (1995) appearing in the November 1995 issue of *Nature Genetics*, however, did not support the 6p localization.

An optimistic interpretation by Peltonen appeared in *Nature* in 1995. Pooling these four positive studies, Peltonen (1995, 665) concluded that they provide evidence that chromosome 6p *does indeed* carry a locus that predisposes to schizophrenia (my emphasis). However, like the authors of the original articles reporting a linkage of schizophrenia to chromosome 6p, Peltonen is quick to note that all is not clear methodologically. One major problem has to do with the variable diagnostic definitions for schizophrenia used by the different research teams. Generally, each of the investigating teams used somewhat different diagnostic inclusion criteria, though several employed two or three different categories simultaneously, seeking the strongest results (in terms of lod scores). All utilize *The Diagnostic and Statistical Manual of Mental Disorders*, third edition revised (DSM-III-R) (or roughly equivalent) diagnoses and related instruments. What most of the teams call a "narrow" definition of schizophrenia includes DSM-III-R schizophrenia and also schizoaffective disorder (Antonarakis et al. 1995, 236). An "intermediate" definition is typically more inclusive and adds to the narrow definition schizotypal personality disorder and also (in the case of Straub et al. 1995, 287–288) all other nonaffective psychotic disorders (that is, schizophreniform disorder, delusional disorder, atypical psychosis, and good-outcome SAD). The "broad" category of Straub et al. adds to this intermediate category mood incongruent and mood congruent psychotic affective illness; and paranoid, avoidant, and schizoid personality disorder (Straub et al. 1995, 288). Straub et al. found their strongest links using this broad definition of the complex trait of schizophrenia and much weaker links using stricter criteria. Other research teams, however, utilized the narrow definition and obtained their positive linkage results with this stricter definition. One of these stricter groups noted critically that the broad diagnostic model includes milder psychiatric disorders with *questionable genetic relatedness* to schizophrenia (Schwab et al. 1995, 326) (my emphasis).[7]

In addition to disagreeing over which cases of the complex traits of schizophrenia should be counted, the research teams diverged in the type of inheritance model they found in their populations (i.e., whether the gene was dominant, recessive, etc.). Several different models were tested by each of the teams, with Straub et al. as well as Schwab et al. obtaining their best results assuming a dominant gene model. In contrast, Antonarakis et al. found that a recessive gene model produced the most significant lod scores. The implications of these different diagnostic approaches and different genetic models are addressed later, but readers should keep in mind that there are many points where the interpretation of the data can be manipulated to achieve more statistically significant results. This is not meant to hint at any fraud or data manipulation in these studies, but merely to point out that there is much that is methodologically less than well constrained in psychiatric genetics and also more generally in complex-trait genetics. Leading geneticists have recognized this as a methodological problem and have begun to advance new criteria for research design and the reporting of "significant" results. For example, Lander and Kruglyak's (1995) article also proposes that the observed *P* values (which can unambiguously be related to lod scores) should be multiplied by the number of inheritance models (thus decreasing the significance level), but this assumes independence—a condition not often satisfied. Correlated phenotypes also require a correction to decrease statistical significance, but it is difficult to articulate appropriate guidelines for this correction. These authors argue strongly for computationally intensive simulation studies and for importance sampling to assess these effects.

A Novelty-Seeking Gene

Another recent discovery suggests the existence of a novelty-seeking gene in a quite diverse set of populations. Though novelty-seeking behavior is prima facie quite distinct from concerns about a serious disorder such as schizophrenia, Cloninger and his colleagues (1996) speculated that a better understanding of such personality genes may give us the best purchase on disorders such as schizophrenia.

Several research programs in human behavioral genetics have proposed that fairly general emotional and cognitive features have a substantial genetic component. Jerome Kagan (1994) recently summarized his investigation into temperament in his book *Galen's Prophecy,* in which he traces back to Galen of Pergamon the idea that much of the variation in human behavior is due to difference in temperament types. Bouchard, in his brief review article (1994), cites Darwin as the source of this view. In *Behavioral Genetics: A Primer,* Robert Plomin and his co-authors cite studies supporting the view that two "superfactor" personality traits—extraversion and neuroticism—with heritabilities of 0.46 and 0.51, respectively, cut across many personality traits (Plomin et al. 1990, 1994).[8]

One of the major contributors to this area, Robert Cloninger, designed what is termed a *tridimensional personality questionnaire* (TPQ) to measure four domains of temperament (Cloninger et al. 1993). These four domains are novelty seeking, harm avoidance, reward dependance, and persistence. These dimensions of temperament were hypothesized to be biologically based on distinct chemical and genetic elements, with novelty seeking, for example, positively related to the neurotransmitter dopamine. Those scoring higher on the TPQ novelty-seeking scale were characterized as impulsive, exploratory, fickle, excitable, quick-tempered, and extravagant, whereas those who scored lower than average tended to be reflective, rigid, loyal, stoic, slow-tempered, and frugal (Ebstein et al. 1996, 78).

The January 1996 issue of *Nature Genetics* carried two articles reporting a confirmation of Cloninger's prediction regarding novelty seeking. The first article by a group based in Israel and led by Ebstein, reports a statistically significant association between the personality trait of novelty seeking as measured by Cloninger's TPQ and a long allele (L) of the human D4 dopamine receptor gene known as D4DR. A second group involving Benjamin at the National Institute of Mental Health (NIMH) as well as Dean Hamer from the National Cancer Institute replicated the Ebstein et al. study. To assess personality traits, Benjamin et al. (1996) used a different but related measuring instrument known as the NEO personality inventory. (The original model was a three-factor model containing neuroticism, extraversion, and openness to experience, the origin of the acronym NEO; see McCrae and Costa [1990, v–vi].) This study also found a statistically significant relation of novelty seeking to the long allele of D4DR using a mapping between the NEO instrument and the TPQ questionnaire.

Whereas all the studies on schizophrenia discussed here employed a genetic linkage approach to finding a schizophrenia gene, these personality gene studies used a method termed *allelic association*. Such an approach, as Ebstein et al. note, works best when it employs candidate genes that a priori make "biological sense" and that have a functional significance in the determination of the trait (Ebstein et al. 1996, 79; see also Lander and Schork 1994, 2041, as well as Risch and Merikangas 1996). The source of Ebstein et al.'s "a priori" hypothesis was, of course, Cloninger's personality theory and his TPQ.

It is important to understand that the long allele of D4DR that is believed to be "causative" of novelty seeking accounts for only a small proportion of the trait in the populations studied. Benjamin and Hamer's group is more emphatic on this point than Ebstein et al. In Benjamin et al. we find that "although the mean score for the L (long allele) subjects is greater than the S (short allele) subjects by 0.4 standard deviations (a moderate effect size), the distributions are highly overlapping and D4DR accounts for only 3 to 4% of the total variance." They estimated from twin studies that the broad heritability of novelty seeking is 41 percent and in the families they studied there was a correlation of 0.23 for estimated TPQ-novelty seeking scores in siblings. "*Thus D4DR accounts for roughly 10% of the genetic variance, as might be expected if there are 10 or so genes for this complex, normally distributed trait. These results indicate that Novelty Seeking is partially but not completely mediated by genes, and that the D4DR polymorphism accounts for some but not all of the genetic effects*" (1996, 83) (my emphasis). Figure 3 depicts the subtle difference between individuals' scores related to the two alleles.

Cloninger and his colleagues (1996) wrote a commentary on the Ebstein and Benjamin papers that appeared in the same January 1996 issue of *Nature Genetics*. They make several points that are worth citing. Cloninger et al. argue first that the TPQ approach was designed to be genetically homogeneous, in contrast to the NEO personality questionnaire, and that this is confirmed by the two studies discussed. Second, these authors suggest that personality development is a complex, dynamic process that has many influences on susceptibility to pathopsychology. More specifically, they state that a novelty seeker is likely to develop into an extravert with a mature creative character if he or she is also low in harm avoidance (optimistic), high in reward dependence (sociable), and high in persistence. In contrast, they find that a novelty seeker is more likely to become disorganized or schizotypal if he or she is also aloof (low in reward dependence and average in other temperament dimensions). They add "In contrast to the quick and clear replication of the D4DR association with Novelty Seeking by Ebstein et al. and Benjamin et al., replication of specific genetic contributions to genetically complex disorders like schizophrenia have

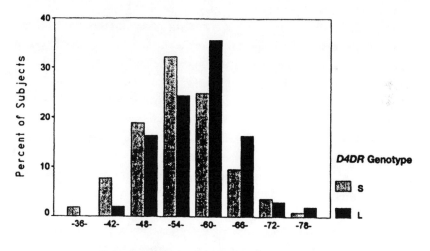

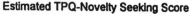

Estimated TPQ-Novelty Seeking Score

Figure 3. Distributions of estimated novelty-seeking scores. The x axis shows the estimated TPQ–novelty–seeking scores separated into eight groups with the indicated median T scores. The y axis shows the distribution in each of the eight groups of subjects with short D4DR exon III alleles (group S, n = 217, stippled bars) and subjects with long D4DR exon III alleles (group L, n = 98, solid bars). (Source: Benjamin et al. 1996).

been elusive. The exponential increase in risk of schizophrenia with increasing degree of genetic relationship indicates the importance of non-linear interactions among multiple genetic factors. When a disease is caused by interactions among multiple susceptibility dimensions, each of which may be oligogenic, then replication of particular genes is unlikely in samples of practical size" (1996, 4).

As already indicated, replication studies have been the Achilles heel of psychiatric genetics, and Cloninger et al. are right to emphasize these difficulties. In fact, although Benjamin et al. (1996) provided a quick and clear replication of the D4DR association with novelty seeking, several other studies have failed to confirm this association. However, an additional confirmation has appeared.[9] Replications or confirmations, particularly of complex traits, are difficult to obtain, partly because of weak gene effects (there are a number of contributory genes), biological variation, and subtle statistical reasons. Lander and Kruglyak make these points eloquently:

> Failure to replicate does not necessarily disprove a hypothesis. Linkages will often involve weak effects, which may turn out to be weaker in a second study. Indeed there is a subtle but systematic reason for this: positive linkage results are somewhat biased because they include those weak effects that random fluctuations helped push above threshold [of statistical significance], but exclude slightly stronger effects that random fluctuations happened to push below [the] threshold. Initial positive reports will thus tend to overestimate effects, while subsequent studies will regress to the true value.... Replication studies should always state their power to detect the proposed effect with the given sample size. Negative results are meaningful only if the [statistical] power is high. Regrettably, many reports neglect this issue.
>
> When several replication studies are carried out, the results may conflict—with some studies replicating the original findings and others failing to do so. This may reflect population heterogeneity, diagnostic differences, or simply statistical fluctuation. Careful meta-analysis of *all* studies may be useful to assess whether the overall evidence is convincing (Lander and Kruglyak 1995, 245).

Cloninger et al. (1996, 4) offer a strategy that may assist with the replication problem in connection with psychiatric disorders such as schizophrenia. They write that it may be more fruitful to map genes contributing to temperament, which has a relatively simple genetic architecture, and can be quantified easily and reliably by questionnaires. They state that later susceptibility to complex disorders such as schizophrenia and alcoholism can be evaluated in terms of the risk from heritable personality traits and possibly disease-specific factors. In this way, they believe, success in mapping genes for a normal personality may indicate a fruitful way to map genes for pathopsychology as well.

Thus Cloninger et al. suggest that there are some simplifications that can be found in human behaviors by using personality genetics that might help to unravel the complexities of less tractable disorders, such as schizophrenia. One question that naturally arises is what will happen as neurobiology advances and identifies all the genes involved in an organism, as well as the neural circuits to which they give rise. Will these accomplishments result in simple and powerful tools that can be used to explicate quite complex behaviors of both normal and pathological forms? We are not even close to this type of arch-reductionist result in the area of human studies, but we are rapidly approaching it in the study of simpler systems. Two of these systems are discussed here to indicate the possible results of complete genetic specifications and their implications for behavior and for mental health.

C. elegans as a Model Organism for Both Biology and Philosophy

Introduction

The cover of the 1995 annual issue of *Science* magazine on the Human Genome Project (October 20) displayed the outline of a human and a worm. The worm was *Caenorhabditis elegans*, or *C. elegans* for short, and its attractive features are the subject of the "centerfold" for that issue of *Science*. *C. elegans* is known as a model organism, which means that it is an ideal organism for learning about fundamental biological processes that obtain both in the worm system and in other organisms, including humans. A quotation from the centerfold points this out, and states: "More than 40% of C. elegans genes have significant similarity to genes from other organisms. These similarities range from sequences shared by all organisms to those found only in Metazoa. To illustrate the potential utility of *C. elegans* as a model system, BLASTX [a computer program] was used to determine that 32 of the 44 human disease genes identified by positional cloning had significant matches to worm genes ($P < 0.05$).... In some cases, such as the recently-discovered early-onset Alzheimer's disease genes, the *C. elegans* gene represents the only significant database match" (Jasny 1995, centerfold).

C. elegans does, however, display some important differences from mammals, in particular, humans. Greenspan et al. (1995) point out that its small size and quite simple forms of behavior make studying its electrophysiology very difficult. In addition, there is the absence of any significant anatomical homology with distantly related organisms such as mammals.

Nevertheless, the relationship between genes, the nervous system, and behavior is probably best understood in *C. elegans*. Though it would be dangerous to extrapolate uncritically from this organism, a close analysis of the genes-behavior relationship reveals some important generalizations that provide a philosophical framework. This framework suggests caution in interpreting behavior as primarily directed by any organism's genes, especially in any "one-gene → one behavior type" sense. To make these points and consider these philosophical implications, some general background on the worm is useful.

Though the organism has been closely studied by biologists since the 1870s (see von Ehrenstein and Schierenberg 1980 for references), it was the vision of Sydney Brenner that made *C. elegans* the model organism that it is today. *C. elegans* is a worm about 1 mm long that can be found in soil in many parts of the world. It feeds on bacteria and has two sexes: hermaphroditic (self-fertilizing) and male. The organism has been studied to the point that there is an enormous amount of detail known about its genes, cells, organs, and behavior. The adult hermaphrodite has 959 somatic nuclei and the male 1,031 nuclei. The haploid genome contains about 100 million nucleotide base pairs, organized into five autosomal and one sex chromosome (hermaphrodites are XX, males XO), containing about 13,000 genes. The organism can travel forward and backward by undulatory movements and responds to touch and a number of chemical stimuli, of both attractive and repulsive forms. More complex behaviors include egg laying and mating between hermaphrodites and males (Wood 1988, 14). The nervous system is the largest organ, being composed in the hermaphrodite of 302 neurons, subdividable into 118 subclasses, along with 56 glial and associated support cells. The neurons are essentially identical from one individual in a strain to another (Sulston et al. 1983; White et al. 1986), and form approximately 5,000 synapses, 600 gap junctions, and 2,000 neuromuscular junctions (White et al. 1986). The synapses are typically highly reproducible from one animal to another, but are not identical.[10]

In 1988, Wood, echoing Brenner's earlier vision, wrote that the simplicity of the *C. elegans* nervous system and the detail with which it has been described offered an opportunity to address fundamental questions of function and development. With regard to function, he suggested that it might be possible to correlate the entire behavioral repertoire with the known neuroanatomy (1988, 14). Seemingly, *C. elegans* is what Robert Cook-Degan (1994) called "the reductionist's delight," but there are problems with a rosy reductionism.

Difficulties and Complexities with the Behavioral Genetics of *C. elegans*

Some serious limitations have made Wood's optimistic vision difficult to realize. I have already noted that because of the small size of the animal, it is not yet possible to study the electrophysiological or biochemical properties of individual neurons (Chalfie and White 1988, 338). Only very recently have patch clamping and intracellular recordings from *C. elegans* neurons become feasible (Lockery 1995; Raizen and Avery 1994; and Thomas 1994, 1698). In her excellent 1993 review article, Cori Bargmann writes that "heroic efforts" have resulted in the construction of a wiring diagram for *C. elegans* that has aided in the interpretation of almost all *C. elegans* neurobiological experiments. Bargmann goes on to say, however, that neuronal functions cannot yet be predicted purely from the neuroanatomy. The electron micrographs do not indicate whether a synapse is excitatory, inhibitory, or modulatory and the morphologically defined synapses do not necessarily represent the complete set of physiologically relevant neuronal connections in the highly compact nervous system of *C. elegans* (1993, 49–50). She adds that thus the neuroanatomy needs to be integrated with other information to determine how neurons act together to generate coherent behaviors—information from studies that utilize laser ablations (of individual neurons), genetic analysis, pharmacology, and behavioral analysis (1993, 50).

A number of painstakingly careful studies have been done that compare the behaviors of mutants with neuronal ablation effects in attempts to identify the genetic and learning components of *C. elegans* behavior (Schaffner 1998). Some of the most interesting recent work that takes the analysis to a molecular sequence level is by Bargmann and her associates, who have examined the nematode's complex response to volatile odorants (Bargmann et al. 1993; Sengupta et al. 1994; Thomas 1994). To give the reader just a brief sense of the specificity of this research, it is important to know that *C. elegans* is able to distinguish among at least seven classes of compounds and react by movement toward (chemotaxis) the odorant-emitting compounds. These seven classes of odorants are distinguished using only two pairs of sensory neurons, named AWA and AWC. Laser ablation studies of these neurons and the identification of mutations in about 20 genes affecting very similar behaviors indicate that these genes are required for AWA and AWC sensory neuronal function.

Bargmann and her associates' work proceeds, as do other studies using this organism to relate genes to behavior, by looking for behavioral mutants. Some caveats regarding the relation of genes to behavior are stated by Avery et al. in a 1993 article: While isolating mutants with defective behavior is one way to identify genes that act in the nervous system, the intrinsic complexity of the nervous system can make it difficult to analyze behavioral mutants. For example, since behaviors are generated by groups of neurons that act together, a single genetic defect can affect multiple neurons; a single neuron can affect multiple behaviors; and multiple neurons can affect the same behavior. These complexities mean that understanding the effects of a behavioral mutation *depends on understanding the neurons that generate and regulate the behavior* (Avery et al. 1993, 455) (my emphasis).

It is almost a truism to point out that a single neuron is the product of many genes, but it is a starting point and might be termed the rule of many genes → one neuron. In the material from Avery just cited we encounter several other similar rules. If (1) is the many genes → one neuron rule, then we may term as (2) a many neurons → one behavior rule. To be more accurate, however, it should be emphasized that these neurons must function in a circuit (which may overlap with other circuits), so (2) should actually be written as (2') many neurons (acting as a circuit) → one behavior. Furthermore, it is a generally recognized fact that frequently genes are not specialized to affect just one cell type, but affect many different features and different cell types (Bargmann 1993, 66), a phenomenon termed *pleiotropy*. This could be called (3) a one gene → many neurons rule. Moreover, in addition to genetic pleiotropy, there is the additional fact that any given nerve cell (neuron) may play roles in several different behaviors, a point implied by (2') (Churchland and Sejnowski call these *multifunctional neurons* [1992, 349]). This complicates but does not make impossible an analysis of how behaviors are caused by the neurons (see, for example, Wicks and Rankin 1995). Bargmann cites some minor neurons involved in the chemotaxic response that are also required to regulate the developmental decision. Lockery and Sejnowski (1993) have identified similar multifunctional neurons in the leech and modeled them using connectionistic neural nets. This rule might be termed (4) a one neuron → many behaviors rule.[11]

Another consideration is raised by Durbin's (1987) observations that apparently strain-identical animals will have somewhat different synaptic connections in their nervous systems. It is not yet clear exactly what is the cause (or causes) of this variation. It may be the result of genetic differences that are hidden at present, an adaptive response to subtly different internal environments in development, or it may be the result of partially stochastic processes in development that Waddington (1957), Stent (1981), and Lewontin (1995) termed *developmental noise*. For pragmatic reasons, we could aggregate these three processes under the heading of a currently apparent stochastic element and add this as an additional "rule" that later investigations may further circumscribe. This might best be termed (5) a stochastic (embryogenetic) development → different neural connections rule.

In addition to these five rules, two forms of plasticity or learning and adaptation need to be considered. Short-term sensory adaptation has been observed to occur in *C. elegans*. Sengupta et al. (1993) note that after two hours of exposure to an odorant such as benzaldehyde, the organism loses its ability to be attracted by that substance, though it still is attracted to other odorants. These authors point out that a more extensive form of behavioral plasticity occurs when the animals are starved or crowded. Water-soluble chemicals that are strong attractants for naive animals are ignored by crowded, starved animals. The authors add that the induced changes persist for hours after the worms are separated and fed (Sengupta et al. 1993, 243; also see Colbert and Bargmann 1995 for additional details). In addition, starving and/or crowding can sidetrack the developing worms into the long-lived dauer state.[12] Thus, to the five rules already noted, there is (6) a sixth rule of different environments/histories → different behaviors, and (7) a seventh rule, environment → gene expression → behavior. These rules further complicate the predictability of behavior; they stress the effect of environment on behavior and indicate the impossibility of accounting for behavior from purely genetic information.

Finally, as if these seven rules did not introduce enough complexity, there is clear evidence that genes interact with one another to affect phenotypes in different ways, depending on the interactions. Some genes suppress (suppressor genes) or hide (epistatic genes) others, and some genes control or regulate other genes. A number of *C. elegans* mutants known as uncoordinated (*unc*)

Table I. Some Rules Relating Genes (through Neurons) to Behavior in C. elegans

---

1. many genes → one neuron
2. many neurons (acting as a circuit) → one type of behavior
   (also there may be overlapping circuits)
3. one gene → many neurons (pleiotropy)
4. one neuron → many behaviors (multifunctional neurons)
5. stochastic (embryogenetic) development → different neural connections[a]
6. different environments/histories → different behaviors[a] (learning/plasticity)
   (short-term environmental influence)
7. environment → gene expression → behavior
   (long-term environmental influence)
8. one gene → another gene... → behavior
   (gene interactions, including epistasis and combinatorial effects)

Note: The → can be read as "affect(s), cause(s), or lead(s) to." The sense of cause (typically as a causal sketch) and the evidence for these roles are discussed in some detail in Schaffner (1998).
[a] In prima facie genetically identical (mature) organisms.

---

display the results of gene interactions (Herman 1988). Thus our eighth rule, one gene → another gene → behavior, where the arrow can be read as "affect(s), cause(s), or lead(s) to." These eight rules are generalizations involving principles of genetic pleiotropy, neuronal multifunctionality, plasticity, and genetic interactions. Like virtually any generalization in biology, they are likely to have exceptions, or near exceptions, but I believe these will be rare (however, see Sengupta et al., 1994 for one such near exception involving the effects of the *odr-7* gene in *C. elegans*). These eight "rules" are summarized in Table 1.

The lessons gleaned from *C. elegans* and embodied in the proposed eight "rules" seem to apply to other biological organisms, including the fruit fly *Drosophila*. Ralph Greenspan, one of the major investigators in the field, writes that his work leads to the conclusion that behaviors arise from the interactions of vast networks of genes, most of which take part in many different aspects of an organism's biology (1995, 78). To this theme of networks involving multifunctional neurons, Greenspan adds that evidence from *Drosophila's* courtship behavior indicates that both male and female fruit flies can modulate their activity in response to one another's reactions. In other words, they can learn. "Just as the ability to carry out courtship is directed by genes, so too is the ability to learn during the experience. Studies of this phenomenon lend further support to the likelihood that behavior is regulated by a myriad of interacting genes, each of which handles diverse responsibilities in the body" (1995, 75–76).

If this network type of genetic explanation holds for most behaviors, including behaviors of even more complex organisms than worms and fruit flies, such as mice and humans, it raises barriers to any simplistic type of genetic explanation, as well as the prospect of easily achievable medical and psychiatric pharmacological interventions.

This network approach should be distinguished from a stronger, quite radical thesis, briefly mentioned earlier. This thesis is sometimes called the developmentalist perspective, although some (e.g., Gray 1992) prefer "constructionist" to describe the thesis, which argues for the inseparability of and environmental contributions to behavior, and for the symmetry of these sources of influence. That is, the cytoplasm is as much a determiner of a trait as is the DNA of a cell. Though developmentalism is an important corrective to simplified versions of the classical behavioral genetics model, as a research program it is more a metaphor than a clear and substantive set of theses (however, see Bronfenbrenner and Ceci 1994). In my view, the molecular approach represented by the examples discussed here moves somewhat in the direction of the developmentalist position, if it is interpreted in connection with the eight default rules extracted from work on *C. elegans*. However, tracing inherited features is not chasing an illusion, as the more extreme developmentalists seem to suggest, and the filling in of the complex molecular developmental pathways will provide deeper explanations of those patterns, not necessarily vitiate them. A good example considered in depth in Schaffner and Wachbroit (1994) comes from cancer genetics and explains the patterns of inheritance in colon and breast cancers with the aid both of recently discovered cancer genes and a multistep etiological model of carcinogenesis. A more detailed discussion of the developmentalist view and some criticism of it can be found in Schaffner (1998).

The eight "rules" presented here may suggest some of the reasons it has been so difficult to find single-gene or even oligogenetic explanations for human behavior. There have been a number of attempts to do so (some of which were discussed earlier) because simple genetic explanations are seen as a kind of "holy grail" for biological psychiatry (and psychology). The next section discusses how some simplifications might arise that may make such a goal attainable.

Summary and Conclusion: Might a Strong
Genetic Program Ever Be Possible?

The search for purely genetic explanations of behavior might be thought of as a "superstrong" or "deterministic" genetic program in the sense that a gene (or a few genes) determines, with 100 percent predictability, a behavior. Stent characterizes such a program as "ideological" and quotes Hall and Greenspan (1978), who write: "The single gene approach to behavioral genetics and neurogenetics starts out with the knowledge that genes blatantly specify the assembly of the nervous system and the components that underlie the function of the cells in that system. Our 'only' questions then revolve around trying to find out *how* specific genes control neurobiological phenomena" (Stent 1981, 164).

If this brief review of the field of behavioral genetics is accurate and the examples representative, purely genetic explanations do not exist, even for very simple organisms. However, in contrast to weaker research programs that seek to characterize only the genetic components of behavior, there can still be a strong genetic program that seeks to identify genes that have a very high predictability for specific behaviors and are (at present) insensitive to environmental variation. These cases were described earlier as primarily genetic, and are the kind encountered in Huntington disease. Based on the complexity of the eight rules discussed previously, my sense is that these types of cases—primarily genetic explanations of specific types of behavior—will be very rare. There are a few comments, however, that may ameliorate my criticism of strong or primarily genetic explanations.

Even within a complex system of the genetically influenced neural networks described for *C. elegans* and *Drosophila*, there are two or three ways in which causal simplification may occur, resulting in something close to a single-gene explanation of a portion of a behavior. One simplification, which can also perhaps suggest points of potential intervention, occurs when a common pathway emerges. This is usually referred to as a *final* common pathway in medical and physiological etiology, in which many different parallel-acting weak causal factors (often termed *risk factors*) can coalesce, funneling toward a common set of outcomes. An example from infectious disease medicine is the pathogenetic mechanism by which the tuberculosis bacterium acts in a susceptible host after parallel risk factors predispose the host to infection (Fletcher et al. 1982, 190). However, investigators probably need to be alert to the possibility of common pathways emerging at any stage (early, intermediate, and final) in the temporal evolution of a complex network that involves multiple causes and complex crosstalk.[13] It is methodologically difficult to determine the effects of factors in complex networks and typically it requires complicated research designs with special attention to controls.[14] The existence of a common pathway, perhaps a specific neural circuit with a specific set of metabolites, might permit intervention by manipulation of the metabolites in such a common pathway.[15] It needs to be emphasized, however, that even this type of simplification really amounts to specifying a "necessary condition" type of explanation (see Schaffner 1998 for a discussion of this concept), against the backdrop of an extraordinarily complex assumption (all other things being equal).

Another type of simplification that can emerge in a complex network of interactions is the appearance at any given stage of a dominating factor. Such a dominating factor exerts major effects downstream from it, even though the effects may be weakly conditioned by other interacting factors.[16] Different neurotransmitters at different points (both temporally and spatially) in a complex system may be dominating factors. Manipulation of such a dominating factor may thus have major effects on the future course of the complex system, though such effects can be quite specific and affect only a small number of event types. Such factors are major leverage points that can permit interventions, as well as simpler explanations, which focus on these factors. Whether such dominating factors exist, as well as any common pathways, is an empirical question to be solved by laboratory investigation of specific systems. This is where the power of model organisms is likely to become most evident.[17] Carrying out an investigation in an organism several orders more complex than *C. elegans* becomes considerably more difficult. One might hazard a guess that the difficulty may increase exponentially with the numbers of genes and neurons. Highly specific single-gene and single-neuron effects in complex organisms are likely to be recognized only if highly homologous and strongly conserved genes can be identified in much simpler model organisms. It will be important, however, to keep in mind the difficulties of determining how such genes and their actions can be scaled up and interpreted in the context of anatomically distinct and behaviorally more complex systems. It is for this reason many researchers believe that the common laboratory mouse, *Mus musculus*, will turn out to be the most important model organism for human types of behavior (Greenspan et al. 1995). Such identifications can give us powerful hints of where to look for such genes in more complex organisms, and they may help to characterize dominating factors or common pathways.[18] As in the behaviors of even simple organisms such as *C. elegans* and *Drosophila,* however, the answer thus far appears to be that dominating factors and common pathways will be rare.[19]

A third type of simplification that may occur is what might be termed *emergent* simplifications, perhaps of the type that Cloninger and his colleagues claim exist in personality genetics. This notion of emergence is not an in-principle emergence, but rather a pragmatic one, similar to the type that has been discussed by Herbert Simon (1981) in connection with complex systems, and by William Wimsatt (1976). It is like a simple gas law being used to describe a very complex system of gas molecules.

It is difficult to predict the fortunes of behavioral genetics, and my somewhat pessimistic comments may turn out to be wrong. Important single- (or oligo-) gene explanations of behavior may be discovered for both simple organisms and for humans. My view is that progress will be made by following three routes, it is hoped in a synergistic manner.

The first route or research strategy is the more classical (but molecular) search for simple gene-neuron-behavior interactions, looking for common pathways and/or dominating factors. For simple systems such as *C. elegans,* and perhaps *Drosophila,* this may work well, but investigators need to recognize that single (or oligo-) gene examples may turn out to be quite atypical, even in *C. elegans.* (Some results not discussed in this paper do seem to confirm the usefulness and importance of this type of strategy in *C. elegans.* See Sengupta et al. [1994].) For humans, this type of approach will almost certainly profit from conserved sequence similarities (homologs), especially those found in closely related species such as the mouse.

The second route is to develop biologically informed connectionist models of the neuronal circuits.[20] This is the route that Lockery (1995) and Wicks and Rankin (1995) are following in somewhat different ways for *C. elegans.* I suspect this connectionist methodology will turn out to be the method of choice, as they (or others) are able to transcend the technical problems of single neuron recording in this organism. This approach introduces its own simplifications (e.g., replacing a molecularly complex cell by a fairly simple transfer function), but ultimately it does attempt to represent the complex details of interneuronal connections and effects of genetic programming and learning on behaviors (see Schaffner 1998 for additional details and references).

The third strategy is to look for what might be termed emergent simplifications, perhaps of the type that Cloninger and his colleagues claim exist in personality genetics. The eight rules discussed earlier in connection with *C. elegans* and *Drosophila* involving pleiotropic, multifunctional, and plasticity effects are themes that should not be barriers to approaches utilizing either a connectionist methodology or one seeking levels where lower-level detail is filtered out in higher-level generalizations. Those rules, however, appear to argue strongly against any simple one gene → one behavior explanation in simple, and especially in still more complex organisms, such as humans.

I think these discoveries, in both simple and complex organisms, tell us that well into the next century one will continue to find an intermingled set of ways of approaching mental disorders in psychiatry (see Schaffner 1994). Genetic results will be partial and will have many exceptions. Chemical, cellular, and anatomical generalizations (including neuroimaging) will play important but incomplete roles. Finally, human discourse will continue to be a vital means of obtaining data and confirming diagnoses in psychiatry.

Notes

1. For criticism of the applicability of the heritability concept in human genetics, see Feldman and Lewontin (1975), Layzer (1974), Lewontin (1995), and Wahlsten (1990) and the responses to Wahlsten. Not all work on antisocial behavior is based on this earlier paradigm. Brunner's work on the MAOA genetic mutation in a Dutch kindred is an exception, but see his qualifying remarks on his studies with this extended family (Brunner 1996).

2. Kupferman stresses that not only do genetics and environment always interact to produce behavior, but also there is no sharp distinction between learned and innate behaviors. Instead, there is a continuous gradation (Kupferman 1991, 989). This section relies on Kupferman's review for its general orientation, but also supplements that review with more current developments.

3. This perspective seems to follow Stent's (1981) proposal to use a more organismic, even ecological, metaphor—a metaphorical approach also found in Bronfenbrenner (1979) and more recently in Bronfenbrenner and Ceci (1994). An overview of the developmentalist program and a criticism of some of its core theses about the indivisibility of genetic and environmental effects is presented in Schaffner (1998).

4. Lorenz's approach to behavior was criticized by the "interactionist" school, represented by Lehrman, among others. For an excellent account of the give and take in ethology, see Johnston (1987), an essay that also points the way toward some of the key themes of the developmentalist approach.

5. There are some similarities between this characterization of a primarily genetic

explanation and Sterenly and Kitcher's account (1988) of "G as a gene for P," though the latter analysis is intended to be both more detailed and serve a broader function than the notion discussed here.

6. Lander and Kruglyak (1995) proposed that "significant" linkage be reserved for those studies that achieve a lod score ≥ 3.6, for complex statistical reasons, some of which will be discussed when problems of replication and confirmation are briefly addressed.

7. The Genetics Initiative of the NIMH has taken an agnostic approach to choosing among three different and increasingly inclusive diagnostic models for schizophrenia, which roughly approximate the three models discussed in the text. It provides data (and DNA samples) on affected individuals and pedigrees, listing the numbers of individuals identified, which satisfies each of the three diagnostic models. See NIMH (1996). I thank Irv Gottesman for this reference.

8. Lesch et al. (1996) reported identifying *a* gene for neuroticism (also described as an anxiety-related trait) that is responsible for transporting the neurotransmitter serotonin, which is the neurotransmitter also affected by Prozac.

9. The confirming study is by Edstein et al. (1997). The nonconfirming studies are by Malhotra et al. (1996), Jönnson et al. (1997), and Pogue-Geile et al. (1998).

10. Bargmann quotes figures from Durbin (1987): "For any synapse between two neurons in any one animal, there was a 75% chance that a similar synapse would be found in the second animal . . . [and] if two neurons were connected by more than two synapses, the chances they would be interconnected in the other animal increased greatly (92% identity)" (Bargmann 1993, 49). This is an important point because it is prima facie support for what Waddington (1957), Stent (1981), and Lewontin (1995) term *developmental noise*. See Schaffner (1998) for a discussion of this issue.

11. These one-many, many-one, and, ultimately, many-many relations are akin to a thesis advanced independently by David Hull (1974) and Jerry Fodor (1975) and developed by Rosenberg (1985, 1994). These authors, whose views I have critiqued extensively (Schaffner 1993, especially chapter 9), infer biological unpredictability and antireductionist themes from such relations, whereas I infer a manageable complexity (see later discussion).

12. The dauer stage of development refers to an alternative developmental pathway brought on by a limited food supply available to larvae. In such a state, *C. elegans* can survive up to three months without food (Wood 1988, 14–15).

13. Egan and Weinberg (1993, 783) use the term *crosstalk* for complex regulatory interactions in their description of the *ras* signaling network.

14. See Schaffner (1992, 1993, esp. 142–152) for a discussion of this type of problem.

15. It might be that a focus only on common pathways could lead to an overly

simplistic, reactive, and reductionistic approach to health care, and to a downgrading of more complex risk factor types of influences. For cautionary comments along these lines, see Rose (1995).

16. It is possible that some of the work on temperament might reflect such a dominating factor or gene, or it may be that this is such a broad phenotype that generalizations in this area reflect many different factors. See Kagan (1994) for an account of this research area.

17. I thank Sally Moody for the suggestion that this point needs emphasis here.

18. A good example of the utility of model organisms is the discovery of a DNA repair gene in humans, hMSH2, that is strikingly similar to the MutS gene in *Escherichia coli* and to the MSH2 gene in the eukaryotic yeast *Saccharomyces cerevesiae*. See Schaffner and Wachbroit (1994) for a discussion.

19. Bargmann takes a more optimistic view and believes not only that dominating factors will become evident as research proceeds but that "dominant genes will be quite common in behavior once we succeed in breaking behavior down into small precisely defined components" (pers. comm., August 1995).

20. See Gardner (1993) for some recent examples of such an approach.

References

Andrews, L. B., and D. Nelkin. 1996. *The Bell Curve*: A statement. *Science* 271: 13–14.

Antonarakis, S. E., J.-L. Blouin, A. E. Pulver, et al. 1995. Schizophrenia susceptibility and chromosome 6p24–22. *Nat. Gen.* 11: 23–236.

Avery, L., C. Bargmann, and H. R. Horvitz. 1993. The *Caenorhabditis elegans unc*-31 gene affects multiple nervous system-controlled functions. *Genetics* 134: 455–464.

Bargmann, C. 1993. Genetic and cellular analysis of behavior in *C. elegans. Ann. Rev. Neurosci.* 16: 47–51.

Bargmann, C., E. Hartwieg, and H. R. Horvitz. 1993. Odorant-selective genes and neurons mediate olfaction in *C. elegans. Cell* 74: 515–527.

Benjamin, J., L. Li, C. Patterson, et al. 1996. Population and familial association between the D4 dopamine receptor gene and measures of novelty seeking. *Nat. Gen.* 12: 81–84.

Bock, G. R., and J. A. Goode, eds. 1996. *Genetics of Criminal and Antisocial Behavior.* Ciba Foundation Symposium 194. New York: Wiley.

Bouchard, T. J. 1994. Genes, environment, and personality. *Science* 264: 1700–1701.

Bronfenbrenner, U. 1979. *The Ecology of Human Development.* Cambridge, Mass.: Harvard University Press.

Bronfenbrenner, U., and S. J. Ceci. 1994. Nature-nurture reconceptualized in developmental perspective: A bioecological model. *Psychol. Rev.* 101: 568–586.

Brunner, H. G. 1996. AMAOA deficiency and abnormal behavior: Perspectives on an

84   Kenneth F. Schaffner

association. In *Genetics of Criminal and Antisocial Behavior*, G. R. Bock and J. A. Goode, eds., 155–167. Ciba Foundation Symposium 194. New York: Wiley.

Chalfie, M., and J. White. 1988. The nervous system. In *The Nematode Caenorhabditis elegans*, W. Wood, ed., 337–391. Cold Spring Harbor, N.Y.: Cold Spring Harbor Press.

Churchland, P. S., and T. Sejnowski. 1992. *The Computational Brain*. Cambridge, Mass.: MIT Press.

Cloninger, C. R., R. Adolfsson, and N. M. Svrakic. 1996. Mapping genes for human personality. *Nat. Gen.* 12: 3–4.

Cloninger, R., D. Svrakic, and T. Przybeck. 1993. Psychobiological model of temperament and character. *Arch. Gen. Psychiatry* 50: 975–990.

Colbert, H., and C. Bargmann. 1995. Odorant-specific adaptation pathways generate olfactory plasticity in *C. elegans*. *Neuron* 14: 803–812.

Cook-Degan, R. 1994. *Gene Wars*. New York: Norton.

Durbin, R. M. 1987. Studies on the development and organization of the nervous system of *Caenorhabditis elegans*. Ph.D. thesis. Cambridge University, UK.

Ebstein, R., O. Novick, R. Umansky, et al. 1996. Dopamine D4 receptor (*DRD4*) exon III polymorphism associated with the human personality trait of novelty seeking. *Nature* 12: 78–80.

Ebstein R. P., L. Nemanov, I. Klotz, et al. 1997. Additional evidence for an association between the dopamine D4 receptor (D4DR) exon III repeat polymorphism and the human personality trait of novelty seeking. *Mol. Psychiatry* 2(6): 472–477.

Editorial. 1995. *Nat. Gen.* 11 (3) (Nov.): 223–224.

Egan, S. E., and R. A. Weinberg. 1993. The pathway to signal achievement. *Nature* 365: 781–783.

Feldman, M. W., and R. Lewontin. 1975. The heritability hang-up. *Science* 190: 1163–1168.

Fletcher, R., S. Fletcher, and E. Wagner. 1982. *Clinical Epidemiology: The Essentials*. Baltimore: Williams and Wilkins.

Fodor, J. 1975. *The Language of Thought*. New York: Crowell.

Fraser, S., ed., 1995. *The Bell Curve Wars*. New York: Basic Books.

Frost, W. N., and P. S. Katz. 1996. Single neuron control over a complex motor program. *Proc. Natl. Acad. Sci. U.S.A.* 93: 422–426.

Gardner, D., ed., 1993. *The Neurobiology of Neural Networks*. Cambridge, Mass.: MIT Press.

Gershon, E. S., and C. R. Cloninger, eds., 1994. *Genetic Approaches to Mental Disorders*. Washington, D.C.: American Psychiatric Press.

Gottleib, G. 1992. *Individual Development and Evolution*. New York: Oxford University Press.

Gray, R. 1992. Death of the gene: Developmental systems strike back. In *Trees of Life*, P. Griffiths, ed. 165–209. Boston: Kluwer Academic.

Greenspan, R. J. 1995. Understanding the genetic construction of behavior. *Sci. Am.* (April): 72–78.

Greenspan, R., E. Kandel, and T. Jessel. 1995. Genes and behavior. In *Principles of Neural Science*, 3d ed., E. Kandel, J. Schwartz, and T. Jessel, eds., 555–577. New York: Elsevier.

Griffiths, P. E., and R. D. Gray. 1994. Developmental systems and evolutionary explanation. *J. Phil.* 91: 277–304.

Gurling, H., G. Kalsi, A.-H. Chen, et al. 1995. Schizophrenia susceptibility and chromosome 6p24–22. *Nat. Gen.* 11: 234–235.

Hall, J. C., and R. Greenspan. 1978. Genetic analysis of *Drosophila* neurobiology. *Ann. Rev. Genet.* 13: 127–195.

Herman, R. K. 1988. Genetics. In *The Nematode Caenorhabditis elegans*, W. Wood, ed., 17–45. Cold Spring Harbor, N.Y.: Cold Spring Harbor Press.

Herrnstein, R. J., and C. Murray. 1994. *The Bell Curve: Intelligence and Class Structure in American Life*. New York: Free Press.

Hull, D. 1974. *Philosophy of Biological Science*. Englewood Cliffs, N.J.: Prentice-Hall.

Jacoby, R., and N. Glauberman. 1995. *The Bell Curve Debate*. New York: Random House.

Jasney, B. 1995. The genome maps 1995. *Science* 270: 415.

Johnston, T. D. 1987. The persistence of dichotomies in the study of behavioral development. *Dev. Rev.* 7: 149–182.

Jönnson, E. G., M. M. Nöthen, J. P. Gustavsson, et al. 1997. Lack of evidence for allelic association between personality traits and the dopamine D4 receptor gene polymorphisms. *Am. J. Psychiatry* 154: 697–699.

Kagan, J. 1994. *Galen's Prophecy: Temperament in Human Nature*. New York: Basic Books.

Kupferman, I. 1991. Genetic determinants of behavior. In *Principles of Neural Science*, 3d ed., E. Kandel, J. Schwartz, and T. Jessell, eds., 987–996. New York: Elsevier.

Lander, E., and L. Krugylak. 1995. Genetic dissection of complex traits: Guidelines for interpreting and reporting linkage results. *Nat. Gen.* 11: 241–247.

Lander, E. S., and N. J. Schork. 1994. Genetic dissection of complex traits. *Science* 265: 2037–2048.

Layzer, D. 1974. Heritability analyses of IQ scores: Science or numerology? *Science* 183: 1259–1266.

Lesch, K.-P., D. Bengel, A. Heils, et al. 1996. Association of anxiety-related traits with a polymorphism in the serotonin transporter gene regulatory region. *Science* 274: 1527–1531.

86   Kenneth F. Schaffner

Lewontin, R. 1995. *Human Diversity.* New York: Scientific American Library.

Lockery, S. R. 1995. Signal propagation in the nerve ring of the nematode *C. elegans.* Society for Neuroscience '95 Abstract. Available from Lockery's World Wide Web homepage: http://chinook.uoregon.edu (which also contains accounts of additional, more recent, work).

Lockery, S. R., and T. Sejnowski. 1993. The computational leech. *Trends Neurosci.* 16: 283–290.

Malhotra, A. K., M. Virkkunen, W. Rooney, et al. 1996. The association between the dopamine D4 receptor (D4DR)16 amino acid repeat polymorphism and novelty seeking. *Mol. Psychiatry* 1: 388–391.

McCrae, R. R., and P. T. J. Costa. 1990. *Personality in Adulthood.* New York: Guilford.

Moises, H. W., L. Yang, H. Kristbjarnarson, et al. 1995. An international two-stage genome-wide search for schizophrenia susceptibility genes. *Nat. Genet.* 11: 321–324.

Mowry, B. J., D. J. Nancarrow, D. P. Lennon, et al. 1995. Schizophrenia susceptibility and chromosome 6p24–22. *Nat. Genet.* 11: 233–234.

NIMH. 1996. The National Institute of Mental Health Schizophrenia Genetics Initiative. At http://nimh.sratech.com (frequently updated).

Oyama, S. 1985. *The Ontogeny of Information.* New York: Cambridge University Press.

Peltonen, L. 1995. All out for chromosome 6. *Nature* 378: 665–666.

Plomin, R., J. De Fries, and G. McClearn. 1990. *Behavioral Genetics: A Primer,* 2d ed. New York: Freeman.

Plomin, R., M. J. Owen, and P. McGuffin. 1994. The genetic basis of complex human behaviors. *Science* 264: 1733–1739.

Pogue-Geile, M., R. Ferrell, R. Deka, et al. 1998. Human novelty seeking personality traits and dopamine D4 receptor polymorphisms: A twin and genetic association study. *Am. J. Hum. Genet.* 81(1): 44–48.

Raizen, D., and L. Avery. 1994. Electrical activity and behavior in the pharynx of *Caenorhabditis elegans. Neuron* 12: 483–495.

Risch, N., and K. Merikangas. 1996. The future of genetic studies of complex human disease. *Science* 273: 1516–1517.

Rose, S. 1995. The rise of neurogenetic determinism. *Nature* 373: 380–382.

Rosenberg, A. 1985. *The Structure of Biological Science.* Cambridge, United Kingdom: Cambridge University Press.

Rosenberg, A. 1994. *Instrumental Biology, or, The Disunity of Science.* Chicago: University of Chicago Press.

Schaffner, K. F. 1992. Philosophy of method. In *Encyclopedia of Microbiology,* J. Lederberg, ed., 3: 111–120. San Diego: Academic Press.

Schaffner, K. F. 1993. *Discovery and Explanation in Biology and Medicine.* Chicago: University of Chicago Press.

Schaffner, K. F. 1994. Psychiatry and molecular biology: Reductionistic approaches to schizophrenia. In *Philosophical Perspectives on Psychiatric Diagnostic Classification,* J. Sadler, O. P. Wiggins, and M. A. Schwartz, eds., 279–294. Baltimore: Johns Hopkins University Press.

Schaffner, K. F. 1998. Genes, behavior, and developmental emergentism: One process, indivisible? *Phil. Sci.* 65: 209–252.

Schaffner, K. F., and R. Wachbroit. 1994. Il cancero come malitta genetics: problemi sociali ed ethici. *L'Arco di Giano* 6 (Sept.–Dec.): 13–29.

Schwab, S. G., M. Albus, J. Hallmayer, et al. 1995. Evaluation of a susceptibility gene for schizophrenia on chromosome 6p by multipoint affected sib-pair linkage analysis. *Nat. Gen.* 11: 325–327.

Sengupta, P., H. Colbert, and C. Bargmann. 1994. The *C. elegans* gene *odr-7* encodes an olfactory-specific member of the nuclear receptor superfamily. *Cell* 79: 971–980.

Sengupta, P., H. Colbert, B. Kimmel, et al. 1993. The cellular and genetic basis of olfactory responses in *Caenorhabditis elegans.* In *The Molecular Basis of Smell and Taste Transduction,* pp. 235–250 (Ciba Foundation Symposium 179). New York: Wiley.

Simon, H. A. 1981. *The Sciences of the Artificial,* enlarged ed. Cambridge, Mass.: MIT Press.

Stent, G. 1981. Strengths and weaknesses of the genetic approach to the development of the nervous system. In *Studies in Developmental Neurobiology,* W. M. Cowan, ed. New York: Oxford University Press.

Sterenly, K., and P. Kitcher. 1988. The return of the gene. *J. Phil.* 85: 339–361.

Straub, R. E., C. J. MacLean, F. A. O'Neill, et al. 1995. A potential vulnerability locus for schizophrenia on chromosome 6p24–22: Evidence for genetic heterogeneity. *Nat. Genet.* 11: 287–293.

Sulston, J. E., and H. R. Horvitz. 1977. Post-embryonic cell lineages of the nematode *Caenorhabditis elegans. Dev. Biol.* 56: 110–156.

Sulston, J. E., E. Schierenberg, J. G. White, et al. 1983. The embryonic cell lineage of the nematode *Caenorhabditis elegans. Dev. Biol.* 100: 64–119.

Thomas, J. H. 1994. The mind of a worm. *Science* 264: 1698–1699.

von Ehrenstein, G., and E. Schierenberg. 1980. Cell lineages and development of *Caenorhabditis elegans* and other nematodes. In *Nematodes as Biological Models,* vol. 1: *Behavioral and Developmental Models,* B. Zuckerman, ed., 1–71. New York: Academic Press.

Waddington, C. H. 1957. *The Strategy of the Genes.* London: Allen and Unwin.

Wahlsten, D. 1990. Insensitivity of the analysis of variance to heredity-environment interaction. *Behav. Brain Sci.* 13: 109–161.

White, J. G., E. Southgate, J. N. Thomson, et al. 1986. The structure of the nervous system of the nematode *Caenorhabditis elegans*. *Philos. Trans. R. Soc. Lond. B Biol. Sci.* 314: 1–340.

Wicks, S., and C. Rankin. 1995. Integration of mechanosensory stimuli in *Caenorhabditis elegans*. *J. Neurosci.* 15: 2434–2444.

Wiesel, T. 1994. Genetics and behavior. *Science* 264: 1647.

Wimsatt, W. 1976. Reductionism, levels of organization, and the mind-body problem. In *Consciousness and the Brain*, G. Globus, G. Maxwell, and I. Savodnik, eds., 205–267. New York: Plenum Press.

Wood, W., ed. 1988. *The Nematode Caenorhabditis elegans*. Cold Spring Harbor, N.Y.: Cold Spring Harbor Press.

Behavioral Genetic Determinism

Its Effects on Culture and Law

Mark A. Rothstein, J.D.

Is human nature "fixed by our genes" (Lewontin et al. 1984, 6)? The debate over biological or genetic determinism is not new. In one form or another, it has been an important part of theology and philosophy, biology and sociology (and various other disciplines) throughout history. Elements of determinism are a part of Plato's *The Republic*, Saint Augustine's writings on free will, and the philosophical doctrines of Hobbes, Locke, Mill, and others. What is new in the latest iteration of the doctrine is the volume of new genetic data purporting to establish relationships between genotype and behavior. Although the basic premise of many of the discoveries is not in dispute, there are differences of opinion about the significance of these discoveries, as a matter of both science and social policy.

This chapter explores the connections between behavioral genetics, genetic determinism, and the ethical, legal, and social responses to this phenomenon. After reviewing the recent history of genetic determinism and contemporary manifestations of the notion, I consider how the law has responded to deterministic societal pressures. I conclude that the law has facilitated and legitimated—rather than resisted—genetic determinism. This past experience does not augur well for the new era of genetic discovery.

A Brief, Recent History of Genetic Determinism

The popularity of genetic determinism, like other beliefs about science, has been cyclical. The golden age of genetic determinism began in the second half of the nineteenth century. As Sir Francis Galton, the father of eugenics, phrased it, the debate centers on whether "nature or nurture" is more important to human development. In midnineteenth-century England there was little doubt that inherited explanations of behavior were gaining popularity. Lewontin et al. (1984) observe the influence of this theory in Charles Dickens' popular novel *Oliver Twist*, which was published serially between 1837 and

1839. When ten-year-old Oliver first meets Jack Dawkins, the "artful dodger," on his way to London, Oliver is described as having a genteel nature and speaking with perfect grammar, in stark contrast to the streetwise Dawkins. Oliver's mode of expression is inexplicable, inasmuch as he had lived virtually all of his life in a parish workhouse, with no mother and no education. What explains this phenomenon? Oliver's father was from a well-off and socially prominent family; his mother was the daughter of a naval officer. According to Lewontin et al., "Oliver's life is a constant affirmation of the power of nature over nurture" (Lewontin et al. 1984, 18).

At the turn of the century, Alfred Binet, director of the psychology laboratory at the Sorbonne, abandoned his work in the field of craniometry (using brain size and structure to measure intelligence) to develop a test that could directly measure inherited, native intelligence. The purpose of his first test, developed in 1905, was to identify Parisian children needing special education. In the second version of his test, published in 1908, he assigned an age level to each task in the test to establish a mental age for each child. In 1912, a year after Binet's death, German psychologist William Stern divided mental age by chronological age to establish an intelligence quotient, and the IQ, the supposed expression of innate intelligence, was born (Gould 1981, 149–150). Stanford professor Lewis Terman created a paper-and-pencil version of the basic test, the Stanford-Binet Intelligence test.

In 1914, seventy-six years after *Oliver Twist*, George Bernard Shaw's *Pygmalion* was first performed. Shaw was a follower of Galton, and according to Shaw's vision, culture was not immutably fixed by biology, but nearly so. Only after six months of arduous work and the talent of phoneticist Professor Higgins could an ignorant flower girl overcome the deprivation of her station in life and appear to be a duchess. Liza Doolittle, of course, was a white Englishwoman. Were she nonwhite or from central or eastern Europe, the task surely would have been impossible. At this time, pauperism and shiftlessness—not to mention intelligence—were widely believed to be overwhelmingly or exclusively genetic.

English translations and American revisions of the basic intelligence test, primarily the Army Alpha Test, were used on a mass scale during World War I as a way to screen troops. The findings of the test were "startling." The test was given only in English, and immigrants from southern and eastern Europe scored much lower than either native-born Americans or immigrants from northern Europe. As I will discuss in more detail, these test results helped to sway Congress in 1924 to reduce immigration from southern and eastern Europe.

It is small wonder that genetic determinism is linked with eugenics. If genes determine the human condition (physical, psychological, behavioral, and social), then improving the gene pool will improve the human condition. The efforts at improvement take on two forms—negative eugenics, preventing the reproduction of the genetically "unfit"—and positive eugenics—encouraging the mating of those with "favored" genetic endowments.

In hindsight, the eugenics movement spun hopelessly out of control. The pursuit of eugenics or the excuse of eugenics resulted in mass sterilization, selective breeding experiments, and genocide by the Nazis, about which much already has been written (see Kevles 1985; Muller-Hill 1988; Proctor 1988). Yet, in American culture before World War II, eugenics lacked its current negative connotation. In fact, hundreds of popular films expressly advocating eugenic positions, including *The Black Stork* (1916, 1927), were produced between 1915 and the beginning of World War II (Pernick 1996).

In the post–World War II period, the biological determinism of the nineteenth and early twentieth centuries was supplanted by "cultural," "behavioral," or "environmental" determinism. The pendulum swung back, partly as a response to Nazi atrocities and partly because of the growing acceptance of social science explanations of human behavior. For example, Skinnerian psychology postulated that behavior was most affected by environmental factors. Nurture, the environment, was thought to be more important than nature in shaping behavior and intellect.

In 1990, seventy-six years after Shaw's *Pygmalion*, the popular American film *Pretty Woman* was released. The premise, though hardly original, was simple. Even a lowly streetwalker in Los Angeles could become a member of high society literally overnight so long as she had good looks, a rich benefactor, and designer clothes. (Cinderella required supernatural intervention to accomplish a comparable, though morally pure, transformation.) In popular culture, the pendulum had swung completely from *Oliver Twist*.

The Human Genome Project officially began in 1990. It heralded a period in which claims for a genetic basis for homosexuality, aggression, impulsive behavior, nurturing, and numerous other behaviors was asserted. This has contributed to a resurgence of behavioral genetic determinism that is based on the misapprehension and misapplication of scientific discoveries and that threatens to have grievous social consequences.

The Scientific Evidence

At the outset, it is important to determine whether, as a matter of science, one's genotype really does unalterably predetermine one's physiological, let alone behavioral, future. To some extent, the language and symbols of the debate have been captured by the popular culture and the salesmanship or grantsmanship of the genetics community. Thus, the Human Genome Project has spawned images of the "Rosetta stone" and "the holy grail of biology," and the individual's genome as his or her "coded future diary" (see generally Hubbard and Wald 1993; Shuster 1992).

There is no scientific evidence to support such absolutist, deterministic views of the role of genes, and there is quite a bit of evidence to the contrary. The closest association between genotype and phenotype is in the monogenic disorders, the classical, Mendelian, genetic diseases caused by a single gene, such as Tay-Sachs disease, Duchenne muscular dystrophy, and Huntington disease. Even in individuals who have the allele for a single-gene disorder, such as myotonic dystrophy, geneticists cannot say with certainty whether the individual will be affected, what the age of onset will be, or how severe the condition will be. Huntington disease was long used as an example of a disorder with complete penetrance, but new evidence casts doubt on this conclusion (Rubinsztein et al. 1996; Nance 1996).

Several genetic principles contribute to this imprecision, including the following: variable penetrance (the likelihood that a genotype will be expressed as a phenotype), allelic heterogeneity (the varieties of mutations of the gene, such as the more than 600 mutations of the cystic fibrosis gene), variable expressivity (the range of severity of the condition if it is expressed), imprinting (variations in the phenotype depending on whether an allele was inherited from the mother or father), allelic expansion (the tendency of some trinucleotide repeats to increase in the number of repeats in a succeeding generation), and the rate of spontaneous mutations (the probability that an individual will be affected without inheriting an aberrant gene from either parent).

Polygenic disorders are caused by the interaction of two or more genes. A variety of metabolic and other disorders are thought to be polygenic. Multifactorial or complex disorders, such as many cancers, are thought to be caused by genetic and environmental factors, acting either individually or, more commonly, in combination. As to vast numbers of polygenic and complex disorders, the predictive value of the presence of a single mutation can only be expressed as a probability, and it may never be possible to determine the precise effect of genetic factors with great certainty.

The final area of scientific inquiry, behavioral traits, is the most contentious. There are several scientific obstacles to correlating genotype and behavior. One problem is in defining the end point, whether it be schizophrenia or intelligence. Another problem is in excluding other possible causes of the condition, thereby permitting a determination of the significance of any supposed correlation. Much of the research today on genes and behavior engenders very strong feelings, because of the social and political consequences of these supposed truths. Thus, more than any other aspect of genetics, discoveries in behavioral genetics should not be expressed as irrefutable until there has been substantial scientific corroboration.

Prior scientific assertions of the genetic domination of behavior have not stood the test of time. In 1865 Galton published two papers in *MacMillan's Magazine* titled "Hereditary Talent and Character." Galton began part two of his article by stating: "I have shown, in my previous paper, that intellectual capacity is so largely transmitted by descent that, out of every hundred sons of men distinguished in the open professions, no less than eight are found to have rivaled their fathers in eminence. It must be remembered that success of this kind implies the simultaneous inheritance of many points of character, in addition to mere intellectual capacity. A man must inherit good health, a love of mental work, a strong purpose, and considerable ambition in order to achieve successes of the high order of which we are speaking" (Galton 1865, 318).

In retrospect, Galton's methodology for reaching his conclusion was absurd. He determined that between 1453 and 1853 a total of 605 "notables" lived. He then explored their relatives and found that there were 102 "relationships" among the "notables," such as father and son. The mere existence of so many familial associations meant, ipso facto, that talent and character were hereditary. In my cursory review of the 605 "notables" identified by Galton during this 400-year period, it appears that the list primarily (or perhaps exclusively) consists of white Europeans and their descendants (including John Adams, John Quincy Adams, and Samuel Adams from the United States). Furthermore, the notables were almost exclusively male, virtually all Christian, and overwhelmingly British. This must have been a comforting but not surprising discovery in Victorian England.

Galton also turned his keen eye to the United States. He observed that the "North American people has been bred from the most restless and combative class of Europe" (Galton 1865, 325), based on their willingness to flee their native country and seek a better life in the United States. "If we estimate the moral nature of Americans from their present social state, we shall find it to be just what we might have expected from such a parentage. They are enterprising, defiant, and touchy; impatient of authority; furious politicians; very tolerant of fraud and violence; possessing much high and generous spirit, and some true religious feeling, but strongly addicted to cant" (Galton 1865, 325). It is interesting to compare Galton's "scientific" insights, which are thoroughly explained in the two sentences quoted above, with Alexis de Tocqueville's astute personal observations, which required the four volumes of *Democracy in America* to express.

By today's standards, Galton's methods and conclusions are ludicrous. Yet, in his day and for decades thereafter, his research was considered unimpeachable. Lewis Terman published a five-volume study in 1917. Using the Stanford-Binet IQ test, Terman attempted, retrospectively, to measure the IQ of some of the greatest figures in history. Francis Galton was posthumously assigned an IQ of 200 for his pioneering work in psychology, although Galton's contributions in forensics, meteorology, and statistics have stood the test of time better (Gould 1981, 184).

In recent years, the most controversial application of genetic determinism has been *The Bell Curve*, published in 1994 by Richard J. Herrnstein and Charles Murray. According to the authors, "IQ is substantially heritable. . . . The genetic component of IQ is unlikely to be smaller than 40 percent or higher than 80 percent" (Herrnstein and Murray 1994, 105). A meta-analysis of 200 familial IQ studies, published in 1997, however, estimated "broad sense" heritability at 48 percent and "narrow sense" heritability at 34 percent (Devlin et al. 1997). Some experts, such as Howard Gardner (1983), question whether there is such a thing as general, measurable, innate intelligence; other experts argue, in effect, that even if there is, its significance is greatly overestimated (see, e.g., Andrews and Nelkin 1996).

In his popular 1995 book, *Emotional Intelligence*, Daniel Goleman describes findings from the famous marshmallow study at a preschool at Stanford University in the 1960s. Psychologist Walter Mischel had experimenters tell individual four-year-olds in preschool: "If you wait until after I run an errand (which took about 15 minutes), you can have two marshmallows, but if you can't wait, you can have one and only one marshmallow now." A third of the children grabbed the marshmallow right away, the others waited. When the tested children were evaluated as they were graduating from high school, those who had waited turned out to be substantially superior as students than those who did not. At age four, the ability to delay gratification was twice as powerful a predictor of future SAT scores than was IQ (Goleman 1995, 81–82). Goleman also reviews other studies suggesting that in older students optimism and hope are stronger predictors of success than IQ.

The Bell Curve is not controversial because, as a psychological treatise, it underestimated the predictive power of marshmallows. It is controversial because it is a political manifesto. According to the authors, not only is IQ real and inherited, but there is an innate difference in IQ based on race, with whites having IQs one standard deviation higher than blacks. "Inequality of endowments, including intelligence, is a reality. Trying to pretend that inequality does not really exist has led to disaster. Trying to eradicate inequality with artificially manufactured outcomes has led to disaster" (Herrnstein and Murray 1994, 551). These "disasters" include much of what can be characterized as the liberal welfare state, including antipoverty programs, welfare, education, affirmative action, and other aspects of daily life. R. Grant Steen bluntly concludes that The Bell Curve is "a political agenda masquerading as science, a meanspirited diatribe against the poor and disenfranchised, and a pseudointellectual legitimization of racism" (Steen 1996, 113).

The Bell Curve epitomizes biological determinism, and biological and genetic determinism naturally lead to a political philosophy. According to Lewontin et al.,"the presence of such biological differences between individuals of necessity leads to the creation of hierarchical societies because it is part of biologically determined human nature to form hierarchies of status, wealth, and power" (Lewontin et al. 1984, 68). Thus, genetic determinism is the scientific justification for societal inequality, social Darwinism, and the status quo.

Flawed scientific theories can be refuted by more rigorous science. A more perplexing social problem involves the permissible societal response to legitimate discoveries in behavioral genetics. Undoubtedly, there is some correlation between certain genes and behavioral traits (see, e.g., Sherman et al. 1997). The only serious scientific dispute concerns the overall degree of correlation and the applicability of genetic factors in a range of specific behavioral traits. What, then, are the likely psychological, social, political, and legal consequences of such correlations?

As an example, take the case of alcoholism. Several past and ongoing studies have explored whether there is a genetic component to alcoholism. Assume there is such a component in some cases of alcoholism. Does that mean that, as a society, we will be more or less tolerant of alcoholics, more or less inclined to mandate genetic testing for such an allele or alleles, or more or less likely to embrace the disease model of alcoholism? On the one hand, it could be argued that the genetic component vitiates the moral taint from individuals with alcoholism. On the other hand, the genetic, heritable nature of the disorder may increase the stigma associated with alcoholism; it may increase the pressure for genetic screening for the mutation; it may contribute to individuals feeling a sense of resignation and a reluctance to enter treatment; and it may lead to disdain for individuals who, despite knowledge that they have the mutation, proceed to drink nonetheless. Research to find an association between genes and alcoholism is being conducted at the Ernest Gallo Clinic and Research Center at the University of California–San Francisco (Miller 1994). If a genetic link to alcoholism were to be established, some of the social pressure against alcoholic beverages and their purveyors might be deflected onto "faulty" genes.

Similar issues are raised with regard to a possible genetic link to homosexuality. If we find a "gay gene," will it mean greater or lesser tolerance? My suspicion is that it will not change the way most people view homosexuals. For individuals who are tolerant of homosexuals, it will reaffirm that the behavior is physiologically based and does not represent moral depravity. On the other hand, for individuals who are intolerant of homosexuality, it will confirm their view that such individuals are "abnormal." It also could lead to proposals that those affected by the "disorder" should undergo treatment to be "cured" and that measures should be taken to prevent the birth of other individuals so afflicted.

Complex social questions are posed by nearly all of the reported or imagined possible discoveries in behavioral genetics. Issues such as drug dependence, violence, and personality traits all may be viewed through a genetic lens. Some scholars are even studying whether economic behavior (Wheeler 1996) and legal doctrines (Berkman 1997) are biologically based.

Let me explore one example of the dangers of behavioral genetic determinism. In late 1995, the New York Times published an article discussing the findings of researchers at Johns Hopkins University (first published in the journal Nature) (Nelson et al. 1995) that male mice specifically bred to lack a gene essential for the production of nitric oxide, a molecule that allows nerve cells to communicate, are relentlessly aggressive against fellow males, often to the point of killing them (Angier 1995). They are also sexually aggressive with female mice. The question immediately raised was whether a similar finding was possible in humans, which would genetically account for violence. Dr. Solomon Snyder, the lead author of the study, was quoted as saying that they planned to pursue the possibility that the nitric oxide synthase gene was involved in some small percentage of human aggression. He said it would be a relatively straightforward matter of looking at certain populations, like the mentally ill or the imprisoned, to screen for defects in the gene.

At a time when there is justifiably widespread concern about violence, the reductionist and determinist view that a single gene is responsible for some percentage of violence, and that the mutation can be screened for, is very appealing. However, it is seductively misleading and threatening. On the basis of a single study on rodents, the researchers were apparently prepared to test their findings on the most vulnerable groups, seemingly without concern for the ethical and social issues raised by such research, and ignorant of the strict limitations on research involving prisoners and individuals who lack the mental capacity to give informed consent.

Not long after the *Nature* article, a much less publicized article appeared in the *Journal of the American Medical Association* (Needleman et al. 1996). The article reported a study of 800 boys attending public schools in Pittsburgh. According to the authors, the leading predictor of aggressiveness and delinquency in the boys studied was the level of lead in their bodies, which was attributable to environmental pollution, ingestion of lead, and other sources. Apparently environmental causes of violence, even those subject to remediation, are less exciting to the public than purported genetic causes.

Even for purely physical disorders, it is important to recognize that a genetic prognosis in the absence of a treatment or cure may have substantial negative social consequences. Are we, as a society, going to be drawn into two camps by genetic testing? In the first group would be the "worried well"— individuals at risk of a future genetic disorder who may never become ill but to whom every cough is the first sign of lung cancer or every dropped paper clip is the start of an irreversible neuromuscular disorder. The other group would be composed of risk takers, who, fearing the inevitability of their demise, embark on sky diving and alligator wrestling. And how would you know whether you will be in the first or the second group? As reported in the journal *Nature Genetics* in 1996, researchers have discovered a genetic explanation for risk aversion or risk taking (Epstein et al. 1996). Thus, inevitable behavioral genetics will determine how we respond to inevitable physical genetics.

Should we accept these scientific assertions without asking hard questions? As Dreyfuss and Nelkin point out, the image of absolute neutrality that science historically has sought to project is not in accord with experience. "The history of science is replete with cases where the choice of research topics, the nature of scientific theories, and the representation of research results are socially structured, and shaped by cultural forces, to reflect ... assumptions of particular societies at particular times" (Dreyfuss and Nelkin 1993, 339–340). The history of behavioral genetics also is replete with retracted or unreplicated studies (Detera-Wadleigh et al. 1989; Kelso et al. 1989) and the misuse of established data.

Before leaving the topic of nature versus nurture, it is important to note that not all observers are comfortable with a bipolar model. Theologian Ted Peters argues that the problems of genetic determinism are not eliminated but merely replaced by embracing environmental or cultural determinism. Either form of determinism, or a combination of the two, is fatally flawed in his view, because both types of determinism overlook the theological and spiritual significance of God-given human freedom (Peters 1997). Yet, even free will has been ascribed a genetic basis. According to philosopher Evan Fales, "just as an incapacity to reason or make choices can be (and sometimes is), unfortunately, genetically ordained, so too it is genes that ordain the sort of brain design that, in humans, is a necessary condition for the capacity to reason well and to freely choose" (Fales 1994, 57–58).

The Role of Law

Against the backdrop of often-dubious scientific claims and morally questionable social policy, it is not surprising that the law has not always served as a fountainhead of freedom and enlightenment with regard to behavioral genetic determinism. This point is illustrated by two historical examples. In 1907 Indiana became the first state to enact a law authorizing the forcible sterilization of individuals with a number of "genetic" defects, including mental retardation, epilepsy, and immoral or criminal behavior. The challenge to Virginia's Eugenic Sterilization Law of 1924 resulted in the infamous case of *Buck v. Bell* in 1927 (*Buck v. Bell* 1927), in which the Virginia law was upheld by the U.S. Supreme Court. The eminent jurist Oliver Wendell Holmes Jr. (son of the leading physician and poet and thus eligible to be one of Galton's two-generation "notables"), and who was then eighty-six years old, wrote: "We have seen more than once that the public welfare may call upon the best citizens for their lives.

It would be strange if it could not call upon those who already sap the strength of the state for these lesser sacrifices. . . . Three generations of imbeciles are enough" (*Buck v. Bell* 1927, 207).

Yet, *Buck v. Bell* was a contrived and dishonest lawsuit. The Virginia legislation was enacted to immunize from civil liability physicians who already were sterilizing institutionalized patients without their consent. The plaintiff in the test case, Carrie Buck, was neither feeble-minded nor immoral as was alleged. She was committed to the state institution after having a child out of wedlock, which resulted from being raped by the nephew of her foster parents (Lombardo 1985, 30, 54). Carrie's court-appointed lawyer was the former director of the state institution where she was committed, who colluded in having the sterilization law upheld (Lombardo 1985, 55–57). The price for this deceit was high. From 1924, when the law was enacted, until 1972, when it was repealed, over 8,000 *lawful* sterilizations were performed in Virginia, and over 60,000 people were sterilized nationwide (Smith 1993, 6). In another of the many cruel ironies surrounding eugenics, the German Legal Code adopted a eugenic sterilization law patterned on the successful Virginia Act of 1924. The date of enactment in Germany was July 4, 1933.

In 1924 Virginia also enacted its Racial Integrity Act, which prohibited interracial marriage. A benign eugenic purpose was used to justify a law with obvious racist intent. The law remained on the books until 1967, when the Supreme Court finally declared it unconstitutional (*Loving v. Virginia* 1967).

Although *Buck v. Bell* is considered abhorrent by today's standards, eugenics was widely embraced by "progressives," such as Clarence Darrow, Helen Keller, and Margaret Sanger. In fact, every president from Theodore Roosevelt to Herbert Hoover "was a member of a eugenics organization, publicly endorsed eugenic laws or signed eugenic legislation without voicing opposition" (Chase 1977, 15, 17). On the Supreme Court, all of the justices assented to the decision in *Buck v. Bell,* except for Justice Butler (the lone Catholic on the Court). Among the justices agreeing with Holmes were such "notables" as Brandeis, Stone, and Taft (see White 1993, 407). The philosophical underpinnings of the decision were not only social Darwinism but a misplaced humane paternalism (White 1993; Posner 1992, xxviii).

My second example involves the Johnson-Lodge Immigration Restriction Act of 1924, enacted overwhelmingly by Congress and signed by President Calvin Coolidge. The results of the World War I IQ testing and the statements of leading eugenicists of the day provided a scientific rationalization for the growing xenophobia in the country. Several "experts" testified before Congress that IQ tests should be used to screen out "unworthy" immigrants, but Congress simply limited immigration to 2 percent of those of the same national origin who lived in the United States in 1890. The consequences were dramatic. The flow of immigrants was reduced from 435,000 per year to fewer than 25,000 per year, predominantly from northern and western Europe. The "horde of the unfit" was turned away.

Put simply, American law was not a voice of reason or a shield against excesses in the era of eugenics. Even the Nazi atrocities, including negative eugenics through 350,000 forced sterilizations and positive eugenics through attempts to breed superior human strains, were all lawful under German law.[1] Would contemporary U.S. law prevent or facilitate a second wave of eugenics?

Behavioral Genetic Determinism and the Law of Today and Tomorrow

One consequence of new genetic research may be a resurgence of behavioral genetic determinism. If so, this phenomenon would have major implications for the legal system. I have written elsewhere at length about the effects of genetics on many areas of law, including employment, insurance, commercial transactions, civil litigation, and privacy (see Rothstein 1992, 1993, 1995–1997). Rather than discussing specific areas of the law in which behavioral genetics may be important, I will discuss five general principles of law that help to frame the issues of behavioral genetics and the law.

1. The law has established a unitary standard for determining an individual's legal duty.

In both the civil and criminal law, the lawfulness of an individual's conduct is determined by reference to the standard of behavior of a reasonable person. The hypothetical reasonable person is not the average person or the average juror, it is the personification of a community ideal of reasonable behavior. This is an objective and largely unitary standard (Keeton et al. 1984, 173–175).

The reasonable person standard, originally expressed as the "reasonable man" standard, was first applied to negligence law in England in the middle of the nineteenth century (*Blyth v. Birmingham Waterworks Co.* 1856; *Vaughan v. Menlove* 1837). The concept was soon adopted in the United States (see Holmes 1881, 108). By the beginning of the twentieth century, the gender-neutral "reasonable person" came into use and is now used in every state

(Austin 1992). The reasonable person standard is often expressed as the reasonably prudent person, or some similar terminology, all of which have an identical meaning. Thus both plaintiffs and defendants in civil negligence cases have the reasonableness of their conduct evaluated by whether it conforms to the standard of a reasonably prudent person under similar circumstances.

Although the law does not consider minor variations in the character and abilities of the individual in establishing the standard for evaluating conduct, there are some exceptions. Children are held to the standard of a reasonable child of the same age. An individual's special talents or training are also considered. For example, in a medical malpractice case, the "standard of care" is that of a reasonably prudent physician in good standing in the profession, or if the individual is a specialist, the reasonably prudent physician in a certain specialty. If the individual has a physical impairment, the standard is the reasonably prudent person with the same impairment, such as the reasonably prudent person with blindness. Note, however, that the reasonable person standard generally has not been adjusted for mental impairments or behavioral shortcomings. These matters historically were assumed to be impossible to assess accurately. Moreover, excusing the conduct of people because of their asserted inability to conform to the reasonable person standard was seen as an invitation to fraud.

The criminal law also recognizes a version of the reasonable person standard. Criminal negligence is defined by reference to a reasonable person. In cases where a murder has been committed in a moment of passion, a reasonable person standard is used to determine whether the circumstances would cause such a reaction. If so, then the charge of murder is reduced to voluntary manslaughter (Model Penal Code 1996).

There are three main rationales for the reasonable person standard. First, the required conduct of the individual and the outcomes of cases are more predictable. Second, having a unitary, objective standard allows individuals to have reasonable expectations about the behavior of others (Seidelson 1981). Third, it is easier for juries to apply; it can adapt and change over time; and it does not need detailed codification.

Inherent in the application of the reasonable person standard is that it is impossible to ascertain the precise cognitive, physical, or behavioral abilities of the individuals in any given legal proceeding. Notwithstanding this established legal principle, suppose precise evaluation of individual characteristics were possible—or even were believed to be possible. Suppose an expert witness on behavioral genetics were prepared to testify about the innate capability of a specific individual in a civil or criminal proceeding. Would this matter? Should it?

Philosopher Dan Brock frames the issue in the following way (Brock 1992, 16): "If a person's genetic structure is a principal cause of behavior and that genetic structure is completely beyond the individual's control, can an individual justifiably be held responsible for the resultant behavior?" It is not clear whether or how behavioral genetic discoveries and claims will affect the law's fundamental assumptions about individuals as responsible agents (Hart 1968). If the unitary standard were replaced with a more subjective standard, it would cause a significant change in the law's view of the bounds of individual conduct.

2. *The adversary system requires lawyers to present all possible arguments on behalf of their clients, especially in criminal cases.*

The adversary system of adjudicating lawsuits was transported to the American colonies from England (Landsman 1983). It can be traced to two Renaissance ideas: (1) the attempt to use reason to understand the world (Sward 1988/1989); and (2) the concern for human dignity, whereby individuals on trial should have a wide range of defenses available in attempting to avoid conviction (Schwartz 1983).

The adversary system uses a partisan presentation of the evidence, a largely passive judge, a neutral jury, and a structured trial format. The lawyer's role in both criminal and civil cases is not to determine the truth; the truth will be decided by the impartial trier of fact—either the judge or jury. The lawyer's role is to be the zealous advocate of the position of his or her client (Rifkind 1975). Overreaching, implausible, or untruthful assertions by either side are exposed through the cross-examination of witnesses and the presentation of contrary evidence. Theoretically, this system not only uncovers the truth, but it results in popular support for the judicial system because parties called to the bar of justice have a chance to present all of their arguments (Stier and Greene 1990, 9–10).

Trial lawyers are not merely permitted to be zealous advocates, they are *required* to do so by legal ethics. The Model Rules of Professional Conduct state that a lawyer "has a duty to use legal procedure for the fullest benefits of the client's cause" (Model Rules 1996). The lawyer is duty bound to make any lawful argument in support of the client's position "without regard to [the lawyer's] professional opinion as to the likelihood that the construction will ultimately prevail" (Model Code 1996), so long as the argument is not frivolous (Model Code of Professional Responsibility Ethical Consideration 7-4, 1996). In criminal cases, even frivolous arguments may be asserted, the only limitation being that a lawyer may not offer perjured testimony (Model Rules 1996, Rule 3.3). During the postconviction, sentencing phase of a criminal case, defendants are given even wider leeway in presenting mitigating evidence.

Innovative scientific assertions come within the "zealous advocacy" principle in criminal cases. One example involves the use of the postpartum psychosis defense in at least twelve U.S. cases in which mothers were accused of murdering their infants. In most of the cases, the women were found not guilty by reason of insanity or received light sentences (Brusca 1990), although it is not clear what weight, if any, was given the defense. Premenstrual syndrome (Solomon 1995; Turk 1997) and post-traumatic stress syndrome (Burke and Nixon 1994) also have been asserted as defenses.

For many individuals, the zealous advocacy standard for presenting novel defenses was stretched to the breaking point by the "Twinkie defense" in the murder trial of Dan White, a former San Francisco supervisor charged with murdering Mayor George Moscone and supervisor Harvey Milk in 1978. At trial, forensic psychiatrist Dr. Martin Blinder, then an assistant clinical professor at the University of San Francisco Medical School, testified that the junk food eaten by White could have affected his decision to shoot the victims. After White was convicted merely of voluntary manslaughter, the California legislature amended the penal code to limit defense attorneys' right to offer such evidence (*San Francisco Chronicle* 1996).

In civil cases, such as personal injury litigation, plaintiffs often have a difficult time proving causation—that their injury was caused by the unlawful act of the defendant. Using what detractors have termed *junk science* or *liability science* (Huber 1991), scientific experts have pushed the frontiers of scientific thinking in asserting that, for example, a particular environmental exposure, pharmaceutical product, or medical device resulted in a particular harm to the plaintiff.

Because of the adversary system, it is virtually certain that parties in both criminal and civil cases will assert behavioral genetic arguments well before there is general support for such views in the scientific community (see Chapter 6). These arguments are particularly appealing in criminal cases because they can be used to prove that the defendant was compelled to commit the act by uncontrollable genetic factors.

3. Judges and juries have little, if any, expertise in evaluating scientific claims.

If the adversary system encourages—indeed demands—that lawyers zealously advocate unproven scientific theories on behalf of their clients, the next important question is: "How will judges and juries view this evidence?" By all indications, both judges and juries are ill prepared to evaluate the validity of novel scientific assertions, and juries are likely to give too much credence to such arguments.

The initial problem faced by a lawyer in trying to introduce scientific evidence is persuading the court that the proffered evidence is admissible. In an influential 1923 decision, *Frye v. United States* (*Frye v. United States* 1923), the court held that scientific evidence is admissible if it is generally accepted as valid by the scientific community.

The so-called *Frye* test lasted for seventy years, until the Supreme Court's 1993 decision in *Daubert v. Merrell Dow Pharmaceuticals, Inc.* (1993). The Court held that *Frye* did not survive the enactment of the Federal Rules of Evidence in 1975. Under the Federal Rules, judges cannot defer to the scientific community's acceptance of the evidence in question. Instead, judges are required to make an independent determination of the reliability and probative value of the evidence.

Judges must determine "whether the reasoning or methodology underlying the testimony is scientifically valid" (*Daubert v. Merrell Dow Pharmaceuticals, Inc.* 1993, 595 n. 12). This is composed of four factors: (1) whether the theory or techniques can be or have been tested; (2) the extent to which there has been peer review and publication of the theory or techniques; (3) the known or potential error rate and the existence and maintenance of standards controlling the technique's operation; and (4) the general acceptance of the methodology or technique in the scientific community (*Daubert v. Merrell Dow Pharmaceuticals, Inc.* 1993, 593–595).

Although there is some disagreement among judges and scholars, most believe that *Daubert*, at least in theory, made it easier to get scientific evidence admitted into court (Capron 1996; Kesan 1997). There is no dispute, however, that *Daubert* made things more difficult for trial court judges. According to Judge Jack Weinstein of the U.S. District Court for the Eastern District of New

York: "Many federal judges believe *Daubert* made their lives more difficult. They are going to have to give a more reasoned statement about why they are letting in evidence. They can't do it on a rubber-stamp basis the way some of them did it in the past. . . . After all, we're not scientists. We're in the strange territory and we want to do the best we can" (Sherman 1993, 3).

Although *Daubert* is not binding on state courts, many state courts have adopted the approach of requiring a more active role for trial court judges in deciding admissibility. At the least, the new responsibilities have caused state court judges to diversify their reading materials to include scientific works. Yet, according to one state court judge, both trial and appellate judges "tend to have no particular training in statistical analysis as it relates to scientific research, unless they worked through doctoral programs in science before making the career switch to law" (Gless 1995, 263). In fact, "they tend to be scientifically ignorant, which means they are not acquainted, let alone conversant, with scientific practice or language" (Gless 1995, 263). To increase the scientific acumen of judges, state and federal court administrators have begun programs of scientific education (Note 1997) as well as publication of manuals on scientific evidence (Federal Judicial Center 1994). It is not clear how successful these efforts have been.

If efforts are under way to educate judges about scientific methodology, no such efforts are being contemplated with respect to jurors. Indeed, the Anglo-American tradition of a lay jury is based on the premise that jurors should be average members of the community and should not have special expertise. Jurors with expertise in the matters at issue are generally dismissed during jury selection, because lawyers are concerned that the other jurors will defer to the single knowledgeable juror, thereby negating the whole purpose of a jury (see generally Cecil et al. 1991).

Jurors' lack of scientific expertise has resulted in a demonstrated inability to comprehend scientific evidence. Nevertheless, several studies have documented that jurors tend to put great credence in expert testimony, even though they do not understand it (Broyles 1996). A key factor is the persuasiveness of the expert presenting the testimony.

The factors discussed above produce the following results: The adversary system demands that lawyers introduce scientific evidence that may not have been rigorously tested; judges without scientific expertise must decide whether the methodology and theories have a valid scientific basis; novel scientific evidence is increasingly admissible; and juries often give great credence to the evidence even though they usually do not understand it, so long as the expert appears knowledgeable. There is no reason why behavioral genetic information also would not fit this pattern.

4. The law encourages risk-averse behavior.

If lawyers are required by legal ethics and encouraged by financial incentives to assert all possible claims for their clients, unproven scientific evidence increasingly is admitted into evidence, and judges and juries generally lack the expertise to evaluate the evidence critically, what are the effects? Obviously, one effect in personal injury litigation could be to establish the liability of a particular defendant. Another potential consequence is to create a generalized state of risk aversion among other possible defendants.

The concept of "defensive medicine" has been widely discussed (see Office of Technology Assessment 1994). It is difficult to quantify the extent or the effects of medical practices designed primarily to avoid malpractice litigation. Yet, this is merely one manifestation of risk-averse behavior caused by concern for tort liability. Other examples include companies discontinuing the manufacture of football helmets, and public swimming pools removing their diving boards. It took an act of Congress, the National Childhood Vaccine Injury Act (1986), to ensure that there would be enough pharmaceutical companies willing to produce vaccines.

In some instances of deleterious environmental health effects, such as those resulting from asbestos (Castleman 1994) and tobacco (Kluger 1996), the evidence of both industry culpability and causation are overwhelming and irrefutable. In other instances, however, such as the harms allegedly resulting from bendectin (Green 1996) and breast implants (Angell 1996), the evidence is less clear. Regardless of the scientific community's position on the evidence, the fear of liability often motivates the actions of individuals, institutions, and companies (Huber and Litan 1991).

Behavioral genetic information could lead to a wide range of risk-averse actions. To illustrate, in a 1994 case a security guard at a Bon Jovi rock concert attempted to rape a sixteen-year-old patron under the stands. The girl then sued the security company that employed the guard for negligent hiring. She alleged that had the company done a background check, it would have discovered that the man had four prior convictions, including one for second-degree robbery. In reversing the trial court's granting of summary judgment for the company, the appellate court observed that "upon discovery of a prior robbery conviction, a prospective employer would be on notice that the prospective employee had a propensity for violent behavior" (*Carlsen v. Wackenhut Corp.* 1994).

No one would question the legal and moral duty to conduct a background check on individuals with jobs such as security guards. Predicting future behavior by using genetic factors, however, raises serious questions. Would employers in the future have a duty to review medical records or conduct their own medical testing to determine whether applicants had genetic indicators of an increased risk for violent behavior? Would it violate the Americans with Disabilities Act or other laws to do so? If behavioral genetic tests were on the market and their use by employers was not unlawful, it is possible that a jury might impose liability for failure to use them, especially in light of the great harms that often befall the plaintiffs in such cases. If there were a single case finding liability, it is easy to imagine other employers being pressured by insurers and the public to require tests of schoolteachers, day care workers, police officers, home health care workers, and numerous other employees.

It is also possible that behavioral genetic information could be required in other contexts besides employment. For example, suppose a young camper at summer camp unexpectedly and deliberately hit another camper in the head with a baseball bat, causing serious injury. Because the statutory liability of parents for the intentional torts of their children is quite limited (Freer 1965), and because a child is unlikely to have adequate assets to satisfy a judgment, a negligence action might be brought against the camp. Assuming the boys were adequately supervised, the injured child's lawyer might assert that had the camp required behavioral genetic testing of all campers, it would have learned that the aggressor child was predisposed to violent behavior. It then could have refused to admit the child, thereby preventing the injury. If the injured child is able to obtain a judgment, or even a settlement, then the risk-averse behavior for every other summer camp, boarding school, college dormitory, and other entities might be to require a review of behavioral genetic test results. Pressure to do so also could come from parents.

These are just two examples of possible liability avoidance measures that could be used for violent or aggressive behavior. A similar response is also possible for asserted behavioral genetic associations involving substance abuse, impulsivity, homosexuality, or other "predispositions."

5. The law has not done a good job of protecting medical privacy.

The recognition of a legal right to privacy is largely a twentieth-century development (Allen 1997). In American law, the development has proceeded along three separate lines: constitutional privacy, common law privacy, and statutory privacy. In none of these areas, however, has the privacy and confidentiality of medical information been afforded adequate protection.

The federal constitutional right to privacy is based on the Fourth, Fifth, and Fourteenth Amendments. This constitutional right to privacy, and related interests, such as liberty and autonomy, have been used to prohibit the government from interfering with personal medical decisions, such as providing and withholding medical treatment (*Cruzan v. Director, Missouri Department of Health* 1990), procreation (*Skinner v. Oklahoma* 1942), contraception (*Griswold v. Connecticut* 1965), and abortion (*Roe v. Wade* 1973). Federal constitutional rights protect against governmental and not private interference, but a few state constitutions also contain privacy provisions that apply to both the public and private sectors.

Even where federal constitutional law protects privacy, the right to privacy is not absolute and often is considered to be outweighed by other governmental interests. For example, New York enacted a statute requiring that an official form be completed when filling all prescriptions for Schedule II drugs, including the name of the prescribing physician; dispensing pharmacy; drug and dosage; and the patient's name, address, and age. The form is then filed with the state health department, where the information is entered in a computer and stored for five years. In a unanimous decision, the Supreme Court held that the statutory scheme was a legitimate effort to deal with the serious problem of drug abuse. It is interesting that the Court relied on the generally diminished privacy rights of patients to support the view that the governmental intrusion was minimal. "Disclosures of private medical information to doctors, to hospital personnel, to insurance companies, and to public health agencies are often an essential part of modern medical practice even when the disclosure may reflect unfavorably on the character of the patient. Requiring such disclosures to representatives of the State having responsibility for the health of the community, does not automatically amount to an impermissible invasion of privacy" (*Whalen v. Roe* 1977).

The second privacy law doctrine, common law invasion of privacy, may be applied to a variety of factual situations. Indeed, the legal doctrine has evolved into four related torts: public disclosure of private facts, intrusion upon seclusion, false light, and appropriation of name or likeness. The first two are especially relevant to medical privacy.

To establish a claim for invasion of privacy based on public disclosure of private facts, the plaintiff must show dissemination or "publication" of private matters (e.g., medical information) in which the public has no legitimate concern so as to bring shame or humiliation to a person of ordinary sensibilities (*Restatement [Second] of Torts.* 1977a). Some parties, such as employers, have been granted a qualified privilege to disclose certain facts deemed essential to their business interests. For example, where work was disrupted at a nuclear power plant because of rumors that the reason for an employee's illness at work was radiation exposure, the court held that the employer had a privilege to tell employees that the plaintiff was ill due to the effects of a hysterectomy (*Young v. Jackson* 1990).

The other important basis of invasion of medical privacy is intrusion upon seclusion. "One who intrudes, physically or otherwise, upon the solitude or seclusion of another or his private affairs or concerns, is subject to liability to the other for invasion of his privacy if the intrusion would be highly offensive to a reasonable person" (*Restatement [Second] of Torts* 1977b). Individuals who are in a weaker economic position (e.g., employees, insurance applicants) often are compelled to disclose or release medical information. They are often placed in a no-win situation, which is not aided by the common law doctrine. If they refuse to supply information, even if they are discharged from their jobs as a result, the courts hold that their privacy has not been invaded (*Mares v. ConAgra Poultry Co.* 1992). On the other hand, if they supply the information, then they have consented to release of the information and there is no right to legal redress (*Luedtke v. Nabors Alaska Drilling, Inc.* 1989).

The third main legal method of protecting privacy is statutory. A variety of state and federal statutes attempt to deal with one or more aspects of medical privacy. None of these laws provides adequate protection, however. For example, in 1995 Oregon enacted the nation's first state law designed to protect the privacy of genetic information (Oregon Revised Statutes 1995). Subject to various exceptions, the law provides, among other things, that no person may obtain genetic information from an individual without informed consent, no person may retain genetic information without obtaining specific authorization, and no person may disclose genetic information without specific authorization. A similar "procedural" law has been enacted in California (California Civil Code 1996).

What has been labelled "genetic privacy" legislation is, in reality, genetic security legislation. The laws only prohibit the unauthorized collection, retention, or disclosure of genetic information. They have no effect on the myriad instances in which individuals can be required to release genetic and other medical information as a condition of employment, insurance, education, commercial transactions, and other matters.[2]

There is no reason to expect that behavioral genetic information will be afforded greater privacy protection than other forms of medical or genetic information. Some constitutional, statutory, or common law theories may be applied to limit some overly intrusive inquiries or unnecessarily extensive disclosures. In general, however, a wide range of substantive limitations in each area will need to be enacted to safeguard the privacy of this information (see Rothstein 1997).

Conclusion

The law does not operate independently of culture, it follows culture. In the 1920s, when eugenics dominated American scientific thinking, it also dominated American culture and American law. How will the law respond to new discoveries in genetics, including behavioral genetics? To what level of legal scrutiny will claims of behavioral genetics be subjected? How will *proven* associations of genetics and behavior affect a range of legal doctrines related to privacy, autonomy, nondiscrimination, and societal opportunities? How will *unproven* or outright bogus assertions be received by the courts?

Legislative and judicial responses to new genetic discoveries will have a major effect on whether we are about to enter an unprecedented period of behavioral genetic determinism and with it, social disruption, or the promised enlightened era of genetic marvels. While history does not preordain the future, it certainly reminds us of the stakes involved.

Notes

1. For a discussion of the eugenics movements in several countries, see Adams (1990).

2. Oregon has a separate law that prohibits employers from obtaining or using genetic information. Or. Rev. Stat. § 659.010 to .720.

References

Adams, M., ed. 1990. *The Wellborn Science: Eugenics in Germany, France, Brazil, and Russia*. New York: Oxford University Press.

Allen, A. L. 1997. Genetic privacy: Emerging concepts and values. *In Genetic Secrets: Protecting Privacy and Confidentiality in the Genetic Era.* Mark A. Rothstein, ed. New Haven: Yale University Press.

Andrews, L. B., and D. Nelkin. 1996. The Bell curve: A statement. *Science* 271: 13–14.

Angell, M. 1996. *Science on Trial: The Clash of Medical Evidence and the Law in the Breast Implant Case.* New York: Norton.

Angier, N. 1995. Gene defect tied to violence in male mice. *New York Times* (23 Nov.): A14.

Austin, R. T. 1992. Better off with the reasonable man dead or the reasonable man did the darndest things. *Brigham Young University Law Rev.* 1992: 479, 481.

Berkman, H. 1997. Applying the law of the jungle: Institute convenes academics to mull law's ability to alter human behavior. *Nat. Law J.* (Aug. 11): 1.

Blyth v. Birmingham Waterworks Co. 156 Eng. Rep. 1947 (1856).

Brock, D. W. 1992. The Human Genome Project and human identity. *Houston Law Rev.* 29: 7, 16.

Broyles, K. 1996. Taking the courtroom into the classroom: A proposal for educating the lay juror in complex cases. *George Washington Law Rev.* 64: 714, 721–722.

Brusca, A. D. 1990. Postpartum psychosis: A way out for murderous moms? *Hofstra Law Rev.* 18: 1133.

Buck v. Bell. 274 U.S. 200 (1927).

Burke, D. D., and M. A. Nixon. 1994. Post-traumatic stress disorder and the death penalty. *Howard Law J.* 38: 183.

California Civil Code. 1996. Cal. Civ. Code §56.17.

Capron, A. M. 1996. *Daubert* and the quest for value-free scientific knowledge in the courtroom. *University of Richmond Law Rev.* 30: 85.

Carlsen v. Wackenhut Corp. 868 P.2d 882, 888 (Wash. Ct. App.), *review denied*, 881 P.2d 255 (Wash. 1994).

Castleman, B. I. 1994. *Asbestos: Medical and Legal Aspects*, 4th ed. Englewood Cliffs, N.J.: Aspen Law and Business.

Cecil, J. S., V. P. Hans, and E. C. Wiggens. 1991. Citizen comprehension of difficult issues: Lessons from civil jury trials. *American University Law Rev.* 40: 727.

Chase, A. 1977. *The Legacy of Malthus: The Social Costs of the New Scientific Racism.* New York: Knopf.

Cruzan v. Director, Missouri Department of Health. 497 U.S. 261 (1990).

Daubert v. Merrell Dow Pharmaceuticals, Inc. 509 U.S. 579 (1993).

Detera-Wadleigh, S. D., L. R. Goldin, et al. 1989. Exclusion of linkage to 5q11–13 in families with schizophrenia and other psychiatric disorders. *Nature* 340: 391.

Devlin, B., M. Daniels, and K. Roeder. 1997. The heritability of IQ. *Nature* 388: 468.

Dreyfuss, R. C., and D. Nelkin. 1993. The jurisprudence of genetics. *Vanderbilt Law*

Rev. 45: 313, 339–340, quoted in G. P. Smith II and T. J. Burns. 1994. Genetic determinism or genetic discrimination? *J. Contemp. Health Law Policy* 11: 23, 31.

Ebstein, R. P., O. Novick, R. Umansky, et al. 1996. Dopamine D4 receptor (D4DR) Exon III polymorphism associated with the human personality trait of novelty seeking. *Nat. Genet.* 12: 78.

Fales, E. 1994. The Human Genome Project and epistemology. In *Genes and Human Self- Knowledge: Historical and Philosophical Reflections on Modern Genetics*, R. F. Weir, S. C. Lawrence, and E. Fales, eds. Iowa City: University of Iowa Press.

Federal Judicial Center. 1994. *Reference Manual on Scientific Evidence.* Washington, D.C.: Federal Judicial Center.

Fimrite, P. 1996. "New Twist in Infant Assault Case: 'Twinkie Defense' Expert to Help Evaluate 6-Year-Old." *San Francisco Chronicle* (June 13): A17.

Freer, A. B. 1965. Parental liability for torts of children. *Kentucky Law J.* 53: 254.

Frye v. United States. 293 F. 1013 (D.C. Cir. 1923).

Galton, F. 1865. Hereditary talent and character. *MacMillan's Magazine* 12: 318.

Gardner, H. 1983. *Frames of Mind: The Theory of Multiple Intelligences.* New York: Basic Books.

Gless, A. G. 1995. Some post-*Daubert* trial tribulations of a simple country judge: Behavioral science evidence in trial courts. *Behav. Sci. Law* 13: 261, 263.

Goleman, D. 1995. *Emotional Intelligence.* New York: Bantam Books.

Gould, S. J. 1981. *The Mismeasure of Man.* New York: Norton.

Green, M. D. 1996. *Bendectin and Birth Defects: The Challenges to Mass Toxic Substances Litigation.* Philadelphia: University of Pennsylvania Press.

Griswold v. Connecticut. 381 U.S. 479 (1965).

Hart, H. L. A. 1968. *Punishment and Responsibility.* New York: Oxford University Press.

Herrnstein, R. J., and C. Murray. 1994. *The Bell Curve: Intelligence and Class Structure in American Life.* New York: Free Press.

Holmes, O. W., Jr. 1881. *The Common Law.* Boston: Little, Brown.

Hubbard, R., and E. Wald. 1993. *Exploding the Gene Myth: How Genetic Information Is Produced and Manipulated by Scientists, Physicians, Employers, Insurance Companies, Educators, and Law Enforcers.* Boston: Beacon Press.

Huber, P. W. 1991. *Galileo's Revenge: Junk Science in the Courtroom.* New York: Basic Books.

Huber, P. W., and R. E. Litan, eds. 1991. *The Liability Maze: The Impact of Liability Law on Safety and Innovation.* Washington, D.C.: Brookings Institution.

Keeton, W. P., D. B. Dobbs, R. E. Keeton, and D. G. Owen. 1984. *Prosser and Keeton on Torts,* 5th ed. St. Paul, Minn.: West Publishing.

Kelso, J. R., E. I. Ginns, J. A. Egeland, et al. 1989. Re-evaluation of the linkage relationship between chromosome 11p loci and the gene for bipolar affective disorder in the Old Order Amish. *Nature* 342: 238.

Kesan, J. P. 1997. A critical examination of the post-*Daubert* scientific evidence landscape. *Food Drug Law J.* 52: 225.

Kevles, D. 1985. *In the Name of Eugenics: Genetics and the Uses of Human Heredity.* New York: Knopf.

Kluger, R. 1996. *Ashes to Ashes: America's Hundred Year Cigarette War, the Public Health, and the Unabashed Triumph of Philip Morris,* 2d ed. New York: Knopf.

Landsman, S. A. 1983. A brief survey of the development of the adversary system. *Ohio State Law J.* 44: 713.

Lewontin, R. C., S. Rose, and L. J. Kamin. 1984. *Not in Our Genes: Biology, Ideology, and Human Nature.* New York: Pantheon.

Lombardo, P. A. 1985. Three generations, no imbeciles: New light on *Buck v. Bell. New York University Law Rev.* 60: 30, 54.

Loving v. Virginia. 388 U.S. 1 (1967).

Luedtke v. Nabors Alaska Drilling, Inc. 1989. 768 P.2d 1123 (Alaska 1989).

Mares v. ConAgra Poultry Co. 971 F.2d 492 (10th Cir. 1992).

Miller, M. 1994. In vino veritas: Gallo scientists search for genes on alcoholism. *Wall Street Journal* (8 June).

Model Code of Professional Responsibility. 1996. Ethical Consideration 7-4.

Model Penal Code. 1996. § 210.3(1)(b).

Model Rules of Professional Conduct. 1996. Rule 3.1, Comment 1.

Muller-Hill, B. 1988. *Murderous Science: Elimination by Scientific Selection of Jews, Gypsies, and Others, Germany 1933–1945.* New York: Oxford University Press.

Nance, M. A. 1996. Huntington disease—Another chapter rewritten. *Am. J. Hum. Genet.* 59: 1–6 (Invited editorial).

National Childhood Vaccine Injury Act. 1986. 42 U.S.C. §§300aa–1 to 300aa–33.

Needleman, H. L., J. A. Riess, M. J. Tobin, et al. 1996. Bone lead levels and delinquent behavior. *J. Am. Med. Assoc.* 275: 363–369.

Nelson, R., G. E. Demas, P. L. Huang, et al. 1995. Behavioral abnormalities in male mice lacking neuronal nitric oxide synthase. *Nature* 378: 383–386.

Note. 1997. Improving judicial gatekeeping: Technical advisors and scientific evidence. *Harvard Law Rev.* 110: 941.

Office of Technology Assessment. U.S. Congress. 1994. *Defensive Medicine and Medical Malpractice.* Washington, D.C.: U.S. Government Printing Office.

Oregon Revised Statutes. 1995. Or. Rev. Stat. §§ 659.700 to .715.

Pernick, M. S. 1996. *The Black Stork: Eugenics and the Death of "Defective" Babies in American Medicine and Motion Pictures Since 1915.* New York: Oxford University Press.

Peters, T. 1997. *Playing God? Genetic Determinism and Human Freedom.* New York: Routledge.

Posner, R. A., ed. 1992. *The Essential Holmes.* Chicago: Chicago University Press.

Proctor, R. 1988. *Racial Hygiene: Medicine under the Nazis.* Cambridge: Harvard University Press.

Restatement (Second) of Torts. 1977a. § 652D.

Restatement (Second) of Torts. 1977b. § 652B.

Rifkind, S. H. 1975. The lawyer's role and responsibility in modern society. *The Record* 30: 534, 535–538.

Roe v. Wade. 410 U.S. 113 (1973).

Rothstein, M. A. 1992. Genetic discrimination in employment and the Americans with Disabilities Act. *Houston Law Rev.* 29: 23–84.

Rothstein, M. A. 1993. Genetics, insurance, and the ethics of genetic counseling. In *Molecular Genetic Medicine*, vol. 2., Theodore Friedmann, ed. San Diego: Academic Press.

Rothstein, M. A. 1995. The use of genetic information for nonmedical purposes. *J. Law Health* 9: 109–120.

Rothstein, M. A. 1996. Preventing the discovery of plaintiff genetic profiles by defendants seeking to limit damages in personal injury litigation. *Indiana Law J.* 71: 877–910.

Rothstein, M. A. 1997. Genetic secrets: A policy framework. In *Genetic Secrets: Protecting Privacy and Confidentiality in the Genetic Era*, M. A. Rothstein, ed. New Haven: Yale University Press.

Rubinsztein, D. C., J. Leggo, R. Coles, et al. 1996. Phenotypic characterization of individuals with 30–40 CAG repeats in the Huntington disease (HD) gene reveals HD cases with 36 repeats and apparently normal elderly individuals with 36–39 repeats. *Am. J. Hum. Genet.* 59: 16–22.

Schwartz, M. L. 1983. The zeal of the civil advocate. *Am. Bar Found. Res. J.* 543: 553–554.

Seidelson, D. E. 1981. Reasonable expectations and subjective standards in negligence law: The minor, the mentally impaired, and the mentally incompetent. *George Washington Law Rev.* 50: 17, 19.

Sherman, R. 1993. "Junk science" rule used broadly; judges learning *Daubert. Natl. Law J.* (4 Oct.): 3.

Sherman, S. L., J. C. Defries, I. I. Gottesman, et al. 1997. Behavioral genetics '97: ASHG statement: Recent developments in human behavioral genetics: Past accomplishments and future directions. *Am. J. Hum. Genet.* 60: 1265–1275.

Shuster, E. 1992. Determinism and reductionism: Greater threat because of the Human Genome Project? In *Gene Mapping: Using Law and Ethics as Guides*, George J. Annas and Sherman Elias, eds. New York: Oxford University Press.

Skinner v. Oklahoma. 316 U.S. 535 (1942).

Smith, J. D. 1993. *The Eugenic Assault on America: Scenes in Red, White, and Black.* Fairfax, Va.: George Mason University Press.

Solomon, L. 1995. Premenstrual syndrome: The debate surrounding criminal defense. *Maryland Law Rev.* 54: 571.

Steen, R. G. 1996. *DNA and Destiny: Nature and Nurture in Human Behavior.* New York: Plenum Press.

Stier, F. D., and E. Greene. 1990. *The Adversary System: An Annotated Bibliography.* Littleton, Colo.: Fred B. Rothman.

Sward, E. E. 1988/1989. Values, ideology and the evolution of the adversary system. *Indiana Law J.* 64: 301, 324.

Turk, E. L. 1997. Note and comment, abuses and syndromes: Excuses or justifications. *Whittier Law Rev.* 18: 901.

Vaughan v. Menlove. 132 Eng. Rep. 490 (1837).

Whalen v. Roe. 429 U.S. 589, 603 (1977), (footnote omitted).

Wheeler, D. L. 1996. Evolutionary economics: Scholars suggest that much of the world trade may be controlled by biologically based behaviors. *Chron. Higher Educ.* (5 July): A8.

White, G. E. 1993. *Justice Oliver Wendell Holmes: Law and the Inner Self.* New York: Oxford University Press.

Young v. Jackson. 1990. 572 So. 2d 378 (Miss. 1990).

6 | Predicting and Punishing Antisocial Acts

How the Criminal Justice System
Might Use Behavioral Genetics

Lori B. Andrews, J.D.

> It is irrefutably the case that biological and genetic factors play a role.
> That is beyond scientific question. If we ignore that over the next few
> decades, then we will never ever rid society (of violence).—U.S.C.
> psychologist Adrian Raine, quoted in Stolberg (1993)

> If it is accepted that genetic endowment determines the propensity to
> commit bad acts, then hereditary traits, which often reduce to ethnic
> group membership, may one day be considered evidence of the
> commission of a crime.—Dreyfuss and Nelkin (1992)

In 1993, a group of scientists identified a genetic mutation that in a large
Dutch family was associated with males having borderline mental retardation
and abnormal behavior, including impulsive aggression, arson, attempted
rape, and exhibitionism (Brunner et al. 1993). The scientists reported that
"isolated complete MAOA [monamine oxidase A] deficiency in this family is
associated with a recognizable behavioral phenotype that includes disturbed
regulation of impulsive aggression" (Brunner et al. 1993).

There were no controls in this study, nor was an epidemiological study
done to determine whether people with that genetic mutation in the general
population have aggressive tendencies.[1] Only five males in the family had this
genetic mutation. Despite these limitations, though, one of the researchers,
Xandra Breakefield, was contacted to be a defense witness in criminal cases
(Mann 1994, 1689). Initially she resisted these overtures, claiming she was
"stunned" by them (Mann 1994), but then, in the case of Stephen Mobley, a
Georgia man accused of murder, she "offered to help with genetic testing without charge" (Curriden 1994). Mobley's four-generation family history was allegedly equally divided between successful businessmen and violent sociopaths
(Nacheman 1995). Mobley's lawyer said, "we're not arguing that the genes

made him do it." Rather, the lawyer stated that if the violent behavior is genetic, it is probably treatable and the judge should know that (Nacheman 1995).[2]

If introduced in a criminal case, the MAOA defense will be the latest in a series of genetic defenses (such as the XYY defense and the Huntington disease defense) that have spanned the past two decades. Such defenses allege that certain antisocial acts should not be considered crimes, but rather, manifestations of illness. In these cases, a person's genetic profile is used as evidence that the person is not responsible or blameworthy.[3] Philosopher Dan Brock points out that "one's specific and unique genetic structure is a paradigm of what is viewed as beyond one's control and for which one cannot be held responsible" (Brock 1992, 30). According to lawyer Maureen Coffey, "the classical Anglo-American conceptions of legal and moral responsibility presuppose humans to be free and autonomous agents who make deliberate choices and who, depending on resulting consequences, are ultimately praiseworthy or blameworthy for their chosen actions. Modern science and psychiatry, by contrast, understand humans to be products of the laws of nature, whose behavior is ultimately understandable and predictable as a function of the causal matrix that governs everything in the universe" (Coffey 1993, 369).

This chapter explores the potential role of behavioral genetics in the criminal justice system. In the near term, evidence of genes associated with antisocial behavior is likely to be introduced by defendants for purposes of exculpation and mitigation. However, in the future, such evidence might be used against defendants and potential defendants to justify a variety of means of social control, such as surveillance or social or medical means to prevent antisocial acts, or preventive detention.

The first part of the chapter describes the reasons for increased interest in evidence of genetic propensities to commit antisocial acts. The second part describes the justifications for assigning legal responsibility for antisocial acts and for instituting punishment. It also describes the challenge that genetics raises for traditional criminal justice analysis. The third part analyzes how courts have responded to purported genetic evidence with respect to assessments of culpability and appropriate punishment, and the final section analyzes how, in the future, the legal system might respond to genetic predictions in the absence of a crime. If genetic evidence can indicate a propensity to commit future antisocial acts, legal questions will be raised regarding whether the state may mandate genetic testing to identify potential lawbreakers, may provide social or medical treatment to individuals with the gene at issue, and may keep such individuals under surveillance or incarcerate them.

The Increased Use of Genetics in Criminal Cases

A confluence of five factors provides the impetus for the increasing use of behavioral genetics in the courts. First, we are in an era when the public and politicians are very much concerned about crime. Both political parties have made crime an issue, and state legislatures are granting increasing amounts of money to build more prisons[4] in the hope that this will reduce crime. Legislators and prison officials are choosing more oppressive means of handling prisoners, such as reinstating chain gangs (Lynch 1996) and creating higher security prisons.[5] Since fear of crime is still rampant, policymakers may seek other approaches, including medicalizing crime by seeking genetic explanations—and treatments. A British reporter described it this way: "Americans, weary with liberal quests for social and economic causes of spiraling crime, are intrigued by the simple notion that some people are born to be bad" (Boseley 1995).

Second, researchers are devoting increased attention to finding genes associated with antisocial acts, such as in the case of MAOA deficiency.[6] Legal commentators have indicated the importance of the Human Genome Project (HGP) in facilitating such studies. Maureen Coffey, for example, asserts that the HGP will overcome one of the current obstacles to use of genetics in the courts by providing more conclusive, legally admissible evidence of genetic abnormalities that affect behavior (Coffey 1993, 389, 395).[7] Lawyer Deborah Denno predicts that genetic defenses such as one based on MAOA deficiency will be admitted by U.S. courts within five years (Verkraik 1995).

Third, there is an increasing belief in the explanatory power of genetics. As an article in *Science* pointed out, "Today the *Archives of Genetic Psychiatry* is filled with the claims that heredity plays a role in everything from gregariousness and general cognitive ability to alcoholism and manic-depression" (Mann 1994).[8] Top geneticists are making claims that behavior will be explicable in molecular terms. Leroy Hood, for example, asserts that "almost certainly there are genes that predict for violence" (Jaroff 1996, 29).

Genetic determinism is likely to be more appealing to the courts than arguments about personal or social deprivation. Susan Mahler points out that "a syndrome is, by definition, more comfortably quantifiable than more amorphous arguments of social contingencies" (Mahler, unpublished manuscript). She predicts that biological defenses will be successful because of "the trend, in the latter half of this century, to equate science (and scientific technology) with truth."[9] This is especially true when the scientific "experts" make genetics seem so deterministic. In an Australian case in which a man with XYY syndrome was acquitted as insane, a psychiatrist testified that every cell in his body was abnormal (*People v. Yukl* 1995).[10] Genetic explanations seem so pervasive today that David Reiss, a psychiatrist at George Washington University in Washington, D.C., says, "the Cold War is over in the nature and nurture debate" (Mann 1994, 1686).

Members of the public and policymakers find it difficult to assess the scientific validity of these studies,[11] and often accept them without question. Dorothy Nelkin and Susan Lindee point out that genetic explanations are readily accepted because they shift the blame from the individual. Rather than admitting one's fault, a person can attribute his or her actions to compulsion—an innate behavior beyond his or her control (Nelkin and Lindee, 1995).[12] Genetic explanations can also relieve societal guilt and give policymakers an excuse to cut social services by deflecting attention away from social and economic influences on behavior (Nelkin and Lindee 1995).

Fourth, a recent U.S. Supreme Court case that lowered the standard for admission of scientific evidence will provide an incentive for greater use of genetic information in criminal cases. In *Daubert v. Merrill Dow Pharmaceuticals* (1993), the Court held that to allow expert testimony, scientific knowledge need not be " 'known' to certainty [since] arguably there are no certainties in science."

Fifth, defense lawyers have incentives to grasp at any straw to get their clients off. In the cases in which the genetic condition of Huntington disease has been raised as a defense, for example, it is often one of a number of defenses (*Caldwell v. State* 1987).[13] In *United States v. Click* (1987), the defendant not only raised Huntington disease as a defense, but also alleged that the jurors might have been prejudiced against him because of his homosexuality and that he should have been allowed to ask them on *voir dire* about their views toward homosexuals. In *Roach v. Martin* (1985), the defendant on appeal raised Huntington disease as a defense, but also claimed that his guilty plea was involuntary, that he had not received effective assistance of counsel, and that the drug he had taken on the day of the crime had been misidentified as tetrahydrocannibols (THC) when it was actually phencyclidine (PCP) (1985).

A criminal defense lawyer's role is to make arguments to benefit a particular client. He or she is not supposed to weigh the risks that the arguments pose for other individuals. For example, a defense lawyer might argue that all individuals with the Huntington disease gene are invariably uncontrollably violent. This may benefit a particular client by showing that she could not have controlled herself. However, it may ultimately lead to discrimination against other individuals with the Huntington disease gene in other settings, such as employment. In addition, prosecutors might ultimately also favor genetic explanations as a way to try to increase punishment by claiming that the defendant has been "hard-wired" to commit crimes. Since genetic explanations may serve the purposes of both the prosecution and the defense, there may be no group within the criminal justice system that is willing to urge caution in the use of behavioral genetics evidence.

Legal Ideas of Responsibility

Criminal law is viewed as a "choosing system" (Brock 1992 citing Hart 1968) in that people are seen as having a choice about whether to engage in criminal behavior. People are seen as culpable when they *choose* to violate the law. This involves both a voluntary wrongful act (*actus rea*) and the mental state to know that the act was wrongful (*mens rea*). In situations in which the individual was not acting under free will, however, the law provides a variety of mechanisms to avoid traditional criminal penalties.

Evidence of one's genotype might be used to exculpate an individual or to mitigate punishment. A person may claim that his genes provoked involuntary actions that caused the inappropriate act (such as involuntarily physically harming someone during a seizure).[14] Or he may argue that his genotype influenced his mental processes so as to prevent him from realizing his act was wrongful and controlling himself. Or he might argue that it is unjust to punish him because his actions are compelled by an illness rather than a "chosen" behavior.

With respect to the voluntary act requirement for criminal conviction, genetic defenses would be unlikely to be accepted if there was evidence that the individual could have ascertained his or her genetic status and done something about it (Model Penal Code 1995). For example, a driver who unexpectedly blacks out and causes a fatal accident would not be criminally liable; however, a driver who knows he is prone to blackouts could be found to be guilty of manslaughter if he has a fatal traffic accident during a blackout (*Carter v. State* 1962; see also *People v. Decina* 1956). This is in keeping with the traditional legal approach, which holds that "the powerful influences exercised by one's hereditary make-up by his developmental and environmental background are not ignored, but the law takes the position 'that most men, in most of the relations of life, can act purposefully and can inhibit antisocial, illegal tendencies'" (Perkins and Boyce 1982, 868, footnote omitted).

There is more potential to prove that a particular genotype influenced a defendant's mental status.[15] If a person's genetic status causes him or her to be insane, the individual can be found not guilty by reason of insanity.[16] There are a variety of legal tests for insanity, with twenty states applying a strict rule requiring proof that the defendant did not know the nature or the quality of the act he was committing, or if he did know it, that he did not know he was doing wrong (Brusca 1990, 1171). In twenty-seven states and the District of Columbia, a more liberal approach is taken, requiring the defendant to prove that he lacked substantial capacity to appreciate the criminality of his or her conduct or to control that conduct to the requirements of law (Levine 1998).

At the federal level, the insanity test was changed significantly after John Hinckley was acquitted on the grounds that he could not conform his conduct to the requirements of the law. Now, under federal law, individuals can be found not guilty by reason of insanity only if they are unable to appreciate the nature and quality or wrongfulness of their acts (U.S.C.A. 1994). Merely not being able to conform their conduct is not enough.

Also in response to the Hinckley situation, the majority of states amended their criminal laws to create a verdict of guilty but mentally ill (Kaplan et al. 1996) to avoid (except in rare instances) acquitting someone who had committed an antisocial act.[17] This newer "guilty but mentally ill" verdict recognizes culpability but allows mitigation of the sentence in terms of its length or the type of facility in which the offender is institutionalized.[18]

In traditional criminal law, several justifications are put forth for punishing people who have committed antisocial acts. People are institutionalized to deter them from committing future antisocial acts, to rehabilitate them, to deter others from committing antisocial acts, to incapacitate them, and to exact retribution (an institutionalized vengeance) (Coffey 1993, 357).[19] If a genetic deterministic view is taken, the first two justifications may be eliminated on the ground that there would be nothing that could be done to change the individual. However, institutionalizing the offender might serve other purposes by deterring others from committing crimes (or from attempting to "game" the system by purporting to have a genetic defense), by preventing the offender (through incarceration) from having the opportunity to commit another crime, and by satisfying society's need for revenge.[20]

Lawyer Maureen Coffey advocates that "In light of increasing knowledge and understanding, traditional yet outdated notions of freedom and responsibility should be modified to square with a scientific view of human conduct" (Coffey 1993, 356). She argues that people with genetic susceptibilities for antisocial behavior are "innately different from the 'normal' person" (Coffey 1993, 356), but that their lessened free will should not make such individuals immune from punishment. Rather, punishment should be based, not on a subjective, moral culpability justification, but on "the legitimate objectives of social control and public welfare" (Coffey 1993, 356). Even though she acknowledges that "punishing an individual for crimes for which he is not responsible in the traditional sense seems to be morally offensive" (Coffey 1993, 398), she feels it can be outweighed by the greater social good.[21]

Coffey's argument will probably be attractive to policymakers, who seem to have given up on a rehabilitative model of prison in favor of a punitive one.[22] Thus, even in instances in which it is proven that the defendant acted in conformity with a genetic predisposition, people who argue that their genes caused them to commit an antisocial act may ultimately be incarcerated to prevent them from committing other acts, to deter others,[23] or to satisfy society's need for vengeance.

The use of evidence of genetic propensities for purposes of exculpation or mitigation comes into play after the defendant is charged with an antisocial act. If it is alleged that certain genes predispose people to commit antisocial acts, the criminal justice system may want to take action against an individual *before* he or she commits a crime. In such a situation, the U.S. Supreme Court decision in *Robinson v. California* (1962) could be applied to limit what the legal system can do to individuals who have an antisocial gene, but who have not yet committed any antisocial acts. In that case, a California statute made it a misdemeanor punishable by imprisonment for any person to "be addicted to the use of narcotics." When the defendant was arrested, he had scar tissue marks on his arm, which was taken as an indication that he had previously used drugs. He was not under the influence of narcotics, nor was he suffering withdrawal symptoms when he was arrested. There was no proof he had used drugs in the state of California, nor was he guilty of any antisocial acts. The jury found him guilty, but the U.S. Supreme Court reversed, holding that it was cruel and unusual punishment in violation of the Eighth Amendment to imprison someone based on the status of being addicted. The Court held that to do so would be akin to making it a crime for a person to be mentally ill, a leper, or afflicted with a venereal disease (*Robinson v. California* 1962, 666).[24] "To be sure," wrote the Court, "imprisonment for ninety days is not, in the abstract, a punishment which is either cruel or unusual. But the question cannot be considered in the abstract. Even one day in prison would be a cruel and unusual punishment for the 'crime' of having a common cold." While diseases in the Old Testament were often seen as punishment for sin (*Robinson v. California* 1962, 669, Douglas, J., concurring), the Court was unwilling to punish for disease (*Robinson v. California* 1962, 674, Douglas, J., concurring).[25]

In his dissent in *Robinson*, Justice Clark pointed out that there was no doubt that the state can punish people who purchase, possess, or use narcotics, even if there is no harm to society "because of the grave threat of future harmful conduct which they pose" (*Robinson v. California* 1962, 683, Clark, J., dissenting). He viewed narcotics addiction in that same category. This logic would allow similar punishment for possession of "criminal" genes.

Justice White's dissent focused on the issue of self-control (*Robinson v. California* 1962, 688, White, J., dissenting). Since the defendant had not shown that use of narcotics was beyond his control, White argued that his conviction should have been upheld. This analysis, too, would have implications for the use of genetic defenses. Unless the genetic characteristic brought overwhelming compulsion, under White's analysis, it would not be permissible to use it as a defense.

The Court in *Robinson* did not clearly explain the reasons for its holding, and consequently, a variety of subsequent defendants raised the defense that they should not be punished for their "diseases." In *Powell v. Texas* (1968), a man was convicted of being drunk in a public place. The U.S. Supreme Court distinguished this situation from the *Robinson* case. The Court noted that medical experts did not agree about whether alcoholism was a disease. Powell had not been punished for the mere status of being a chronic alcoholic; he had engaged in a particular act—being in public while drunk. The Court also indicated that since there are no adequate treatments, facilities, or manpower to aid alcoholics, the use of the criminal process as a means of dealing with the public aspects of problem drinking could be seen as rational. The Court found no constitutional requirement that punishment be rehabilitative or therapeutic (*Powell v. Texas* 1968).[26]

Moreover, even the *Robinson* case listed a variety of interventions that states could constitutionally undertake based on the "status" of addiction—including compulsory treatment with involuntary confinement and penal sanctions for failure to undergo treatment (*Robinson v. California* 1962, 664).[27] "The addict is a sick person," wrote Justice Douglas, concurring. "He may, of course, be confined for treatment or for the protection of society" (*Robinson v. California* 1962, 676, Douglas, J., concurring).

The general legal precedents addressing free will and criminal responsibility will influence how courts deal with genetic defenses. It is likely that such defenses will be applicable only in limited circumstances, in which the defendants can meet a heavy burden of proof to show that their genetic status caused them to not know what they were doing, not realize it was wrong, or (in a limited number of jurisdictions) not be able to conform their conduct to the requirements of the law.[28] With respect to punishment, however, even if a person uses behavioral genetics evidence as a defense, courts may still be willing to incarcerate the individual for the individual's own good or to protect others in society.

Cases Involving Genetic Defenses

The use of genetic defenses began in the early 1970s with the XYY defense. The first XYY male identified was of average intelligence, without physical defects, and not in prison (Sanberg 1961). However, identification of the unusual chromosomal complement caused researchers to begin research on the chromosome types of inmates. In 1965, researchers reported that they found that seven of the 197 inmates in a maximum security hospital had the XYY karyotype (Burke 1969, 264, citing Jacobs et al. 1965). Since the expected prevalence of XYY in the population was approximately 1 in 1500, the seeming overrepresentation of men with that chromosomal complement in prison led to speculation that there was "a strong positive correlation between antisocial behavior and the XYY individual" (Burke 1969, 267).

As a direct result of the research, defendants began to argue that their chromosome type was relevant to a defense. In Australia, a defendant with the XYY chromosomal complement was acquitted by reason of insanity (see discussion in *People v. Tanner* 1970). In the United States, the XYY defense has been considered under various formulations of the insanity defense. Twenty-six years ago, a California court considering the XYY defense indicated that it would recognize a genetic defense if the genetic condition was clearly and convincingly linked to insanity (*People v. Tanner* 1970).[29] A few years later, a New York court produced a more refined test, opening up the possibility of using a genetic defense as long as there is a high degree of medical certainty that the genetic syndrome has affected the defendant's mental capacity so as to "interfere substantially with the defendant's cognitive capacity or with his ability to understand or appreciate the basic moral code of his society" (*People v. Yukl* 1975, 319). An alternative test was set forth in a Maryland case (*Millard v. State* 1970, 229), in which the court held that to show that a defendant with an XYY chromosomal complement was insane, he must be shown to lack "substantial capacity either to appreciate the criminality of his conduct or to conform his conduct to the requirements of law." In all these cases, the courts rejected the XYY defense, although in the Maryland case there was an indication the defense might have been successful if a psychiatrist had been called as an expert witness in addition to the geneticist.[30]

Later, more rigorous studies of the general population found that there was no increased incidence of violent crime among men with the XYY chromosomal complement (Freyne and O'Connor 1992). As a 1976 Washington court observed, in rejecting an XYY defense, "presently available medical evidence is unable to establish a reasonably certain causal connection between the XYY defect and criminal conduct" (*State v. Roberts* 1976).

More recent genetic defense cases have alleged that the defendants are in the early stages of Huntington disease. In one case in which Huntington disease was proven, the individual was acquitted by reason of insanity. On July 7, 1985, Glenda Sue Caldwell cleaned her house and disposed of certain books about well-publicized murders. When her nineteen-year-old son arrived home for lunch, she shot and killed him and then tried unsuccessfully to kill her daughters (*Caldwell v. State* 1987). She told the police officer who arrived on the scene that she was going through a divorce and intended to kill her children, then herself.

Her defense at trial was insanity brought on by her fear of developing Huntington disease and her separation from her husband. Her daughter testified that the defendant appeared sane at the time of the shooting. The psychiatrists at trial testified that she was sane. The jury, too, found her to have been sane at the time and returned a verdict of "guilty but mentally ill" (*Caldwell v. State* 1987).

In 1992, Caldwell became symptomatic with Huntington disease. She won a new trial and on August 25, 1994, a judge found her not guilty by reason of insanity (AP 1994). Such a verdict stretches credulity. If she had not been viewed as insane in her first trial, which took place closer to the time that she killed her son, how does her subsequent development of Huntington disease symptoms provide evidence she was insane nine years earlier?

Huntington disease has been used in other ways to dispute guilt. On October 16, 1985, Luther Erwin Click confessed to an FBI agent that he had robbed a bank of $2,000 earlier that day. At trial, Click did not allege that his disease made him commit the crime. Rather—more innovatively—he alleged that he had falsely confessed to the crime in order to receive improved institutional care for his illness (*United States v. Click* 1987). When he was convicted of the bank robbery, he appealed on the grounds that the trial judge had not admitted his more than 500 pages of medical records, which he claimed would have shown he would rather have gone to jail than continue with the inadequate care he had received. The appellate court affirmed the conviction on the grounds that the medical records were irrelevant since they would not have proven that the confession was false.

There is yet another way in which Huntington disease might be raised in a criminal context. It might be alleged that a particular crime was justified because the *victim* had Huntington disease. A Swedish woman was acquitted by an appeals court of an euthanasia charge. She had given a fatal mixture of pills and alcohol to her 26-year-old daughter, who had Huntington disease (Agence France Presse 1996). The appeals court indicated that by putting pills in the daughter's mouth and giving her alcohol, the mother was enabling the daughter's own actions, and thus did not take the daughter's life. However, it may be that the nature of the daughter's condition also made the action seem more justifiable. In a previous case, a woman was sentenced to prison after helping a man with multiple sclerosis take his life (Agence France Presse 1996).

Consequences for Punishment

In addition to disputing guilt, genetic evidence has been used to mitigate punishment. In France, a convicted murderer with the XYY chromosomal complement received a lesser sentence (see discussion in *People v. Tanner* 1970). When a California attorney who misappropriated client funds claimed at disbarment hearings that he had a genetic predisposition to alcoholism, he was placed on probation rather than disbarred (*In re Ewaniszyk* 1990). In contrast, another attorney, who had been an alcoholic and misappropriated client funds, but did not raise a genetic defense, was disbarred (*Baker v. State Bar of California* 1989).[31] It may not have been the genetic condition itself that led to the more lenient sentence. Rather, the court said that "evidence that the petitioner was not properly diagnosed when he was released from his initial treatment program is mitigating" (*Baker v. State Bar of California* 1989).

In contrast, a genetic predisposition might be used to *enhance* punishment. A genetic propensity for antisocial acts may be viewed as indicating that there is nothing that the defendant can do to change his or her nature, and consequently society might lock the person up forever to protect itself or even use the death penalty. In Texas, for example, a jury deciding on the death penalty must consider "whether there is a probability that the defendant would commit criminal acts of violence that would constitute a continuing threat to society" (Texas Criminal Procedure Code 1996).

Under such an approach, evidence of a genetic propensity may end up being, not a defense, but a stigma. Such people might be written off, without attention being paid to attempts to rehabilitate them. This social trend of vindictiveness is evident in the popularity of Richard Herrnstein and Charles Murray's book, *The Bell Curve* (1994), which has been interpreted to stand for the principle that we should not fund enrichment programs for young black children because they have built-in genetic limitations on cognitive abilities.[32]

A third approach would be to ignore genetic status in sentencing. In *Scammahorn v. State*, Michael Scammahorn was stalking an ex-girlfriend with a gun when her father intervened and he shot the father (*Scammahorn v. State* 1987). He was found guilty but mentally ill. On appeal, he claimed that his sentence of twenty years for attempted murder should be suspended because he had Huntington disease. The court, however, indicated that whether he had Huntington disease would not be relevant to the sentence. "If we consider for the sake of argument that the fact that the appellant was suffering from the early stages of Huntington's disease is a mitigating factor, the court was nevertheless not required to reduce or suspend the sentence for that reason" (*Scammahorn v. State* 1987, 1099).

Access to Appropriate Testing

If genetic assessments were relevant to determining culpability or sentencing, questions would arise regarding whether the state should pay for testing.[33] If the state does not, a genetic defense might only be available to the rich (Dreyfuss and Nelkin 1992, 329). In addition to questions of payments for testing, issues will be raised about whether a certain type of testing is sufficiently reliable or accepted to be admitted.

The issue of test reliability was raised in *Roach v. Martin* (1985). On December 13, 1977, James Terry Roach pleaded guilty to two counts of murder, criminal sexual conduct, armed robbery, and kidnapping.[34] At the hearing, it was acknowledged that Roach's mother had Huntington disease, but an expert for the state and one for the defense determined Roach did not have the disease and found it impossible to determine whether he ever would. (This was before the gene for Huntington disease had been located.) The judge sentenced Roach to death.

On appeal, the court was not persuaded by Roach's argument that his trial counsel should have investigated Huntington disease further and learned that substance abuse is an involuntary symptom of Huntington disease (*Roach v. Martin* 1985, 1479). Since there was no evidence that Roach had Huntington disease, this argument was dismissed.

Also on appeal, Roach tried to gain a new hearing on the grounds that "new evidence" had been discovered. This new evidence was not evidence related to the crime, but was the possibility of using position emission tomography, a PET scan, to detect Huntington disease before the onset of symptoms. There were two problems with this argument, however. One was the lack of evidence that the PET scan was reliable. Defense counsel had provided no scientific support for the procedure, other than an undated National Institute of Mental Health internal memorandum. The second problem was that the court considered the evidence to be irrelevant. The court stated, "even assuming arguendo that Roach does in fact have the Huntington's gene, in which case Huntington's disease will inevitably manifest its symptoms, we can see no way that this fact alone would alter Roach's conviction and sentence" (*Roach v. Martin* 1985, 1474). The court indicated that since Roach had not provided evidence he was insane, finding that he had the Huntington gene would not change the assessment that he was sane at the time of the crime, competent to stand trial, or currently competent. And even though it is cruel and unusual punishment under the Eighth Amendment to execute someone who is insane, Roach had not shown that having the Huntington gene was equated with insanity. Consequently, Roach's conviction was affirmed.

Predicting Future Acts

If genetic predispositions are identified for antisocial acts, there may be a strong social interest in attempting to *prevent* the commission of the acts in the first place. A program of prevention might include any or all of the following phases: identifying people who have the antisocial genes, attempting social means to dissuade them from antisocial behavior, keeping such individuals under surveillance, mandating treatment to counteract the genetic propensity, or preventively detaining them to eliminate the opportunity for an antisocial act.[35] My own opinion is that to the extent society chooses to define genetic predisposition to antisocial acts as a medical issue, there will be a tendency to allow interventions that would otherwise, in a sheer criminal justice context, be seen as unconstitutionally infringing an individual's rights.

Identifying People with Antisocial Genes

Collecting tissue samples from an individual who has not otherwise been charged or convicted of a crime would likely be seen as violating the person's federal constitutional Fourth Amendment right to be free from unreasonable searches and seizures. However, it may not be necessary to actually collect blood or other tissue samples since there is potentially a wealth of tissue samples already on file regarding individuals. Hospitals often maintain patients' samples from blood tests, biopsies, and surgical procedures. State newborn screening programs have collected blood from virtually all infants born since the late 1960s (Andrews 1985). Many states have maintained the samples and few have rules that limit the use that can be made of them (McEwen and Reilly 1994b). The Department of Defense is collecting DNA samples on all new recruits and active servicemen; an estimated 18 million military people will eventually have samples on file (Chadwin 1996). In all fifty states, certain offenders must provide blood samples for forensic DNA banks (Hibbert 1998).[36] In some states, the reach of the statutes is quite broad. Courts have been willing to authorize collection of DNA for forensic banks even from nonviolent offenders.[37] This means that an individual convicted of swearing at a basketball game (a misdemeanor in some states) could be obliged to provide a DNA sample.

Moreover, an increasing number of people are seeking genetic testing for medical purposes. In some instances, such as testing for Huntington disease, that information may be viewed as predictive of future behaviors. In other instances, an individual may seek genetic information relevant to a particular medical condition, but the information will later be determined to be predictive of a particular behavior as well. For example, people have sought apo E4 testing to learn whether they are at increased risk for heart disease. Subsequently, it has been asserted that the apo E4 gene also predicts an increased risk for Alzheimer disease (Kolata 1995).

Whether the Fourth Amendment might protect against the secondary use of existing samples is a matter of more dispute, since an invasion of bodily integrity does not occur. However, various legal and policy arguments can be made against forcing people to learn new genetic information about themselves (see Andrews 1996), information that is not directly related to the purpose for which the sample was initially collected. Moreover, the U.S. Supreme Court, recognizing the privacy interests in information, has held that analysis of tissue samples (such as urine samples) constitutes a search, even when the government already has possession of the samples (*Veronia School District 47J v. Acton* 1995, 2393). A few states have genetic privacy laws that prohibit DNA testing without consent. A statute in Colorado provides such protection, saying "Genetic information is the unique property of the individual to whom the information pertains. . . . Information derived from genetic testing shall be confidential and privileged. Any release, for purposes other than diagnosis, treatment, or therapy, of genetic testing information that identifies the person tested with the test results released requires specific written consent by the person tested" (Colorado Stat. Ann. 1994). Similarly, a Florida law provides that (other than in forensic settings) "DNA analysis may be performed only with the informed consent of the person to be tested, and the results of such DNA analysis, whether held by a public or private entity, are the exclusive property of the person tested, are confidential, and may not be disclosed without the consent of the person tested" (Florida Stat. Ann 1995). Likewise, Oregon has a law that provides that except in extremely limited circumstances, "no person shall obtain genetic information from an individual, or from an individual's DNA sample, without first obtaining informed consent of the individual or the individual's representative." In addition, a Washington regulation prohibits use of forensic DNA data for research other than that related to a criminal investigation or improving the operation of the criminal justice system (McEwen and Reilly 1994a, 951).[38]

Law professor Harold Krent argues for restriction under the Fourth Amendment of the secondary uses of governmentally seized items and information (including DNA) since "what governmental officials do with seized information and items may affect an individual's privacy and property rights as much as the seizure itself" (Krent 1995, 77). He advocates a system in which, in the law enforcement context, all future uses of DNA must be disclosed to and assessed by a court at the time the decision to collect the DNA is made.

Nevertheless, some courts may be willing to ignore privacy arguments and Fourth Amendment extensions and instead mandate programs of genetic screening of existing samples for antisocial genes on the ground that it does not involve bodily intrusion. Since genetic samples from and genetic information about many individuals already exist, and there are few explicit bans on states' use of them to look for "criminal" genes, there is the potential for the criminal justice system to take action using genetic information about potential antisocial acts.

Attempting Social Means to Dissuade People from Antisocial Acts

Once people are identified as having genetic predispositions to antisocial acts, a variety of social means might be taken to deter such behaviors.[39] Currently, for example, there are various programs to teach schoolchildren identified as having high violence potential to act in less aggressive ways. More than 8,600 children in sixteen Chicago area schools have participated in such a violence prevention program, run by University of Illinois psychologists and funded by the National Institutes of Health (Stolberg 1993).

The program is based on research undertaken in the 1960s which found that children who were aggressive at age eight grew up to be three times as likely to commit crime at age thirty (Stolberg 1993). In the Chicago program, the parents are not told the reason their children are being counseled. Instead, they are told they have been selected to be part of "leadership training" (Stolberg 1993). The ethics of such a deception are complicated. Perhaps if parents were told their children were prone to violence they would treat the children in such a way that it would become a self-fulfilling prophecy. Yet, this means that the school is collecting data on—and intervening with—children without their parents' true consent. If the school's analysis of which children were most highly prone to crime was leaked, these children might find that they were later denied jobs by employers who wanted to avoid the risk of crime. Moreover, since the original study only predicted an increased propensity toward crime—not that all of the children identified would turn out to be criminals—there will be interventions with children who do not need them. In the original study, 23 percent of the "most aggressive" group of third graders had been convicted of crimes by age thirty as opposed to 9 percent of the "least aggressive" group (Hilts 1983).[40]

The use of social means to prevent violence is likely to be upheld as an appropriate education program, even though it is both overinclusive and underinclusive. People without a purported genetic propensity to antisocial acts will commit crimes, and those with the supposedly predisposing allele will not. In some states, there will be potential legal actions for breaches of confidentiality or invasion of privacy if information about someone's genotype is disclosed to third parties and the individual is financially harmed in some way as a result.[41] However, most states do not protect genetic information sufficiently (Andrews 1995).

Mandating Medical Treatment

In some instances, social interventions may not seem adequate to deal with purported genetic propensities toward criminal acts. Instead, medical interventions (ranging from drug treatment to surgery to gene therapy) might be suggested. Such an approach will fit in with an increasing tendency to view violence as a medical problem.

The Centers for Disease Control and Prevention has declared violence a pressing public health problem.[42] The *Los Angeles Times* ran an article about the high medical costs of violence, noting that "each year, more than 2 million Americans suffer injuries as a result of violence, and more than 500,000 are treated in emergency rooms." The newspaper estimated that it costs $18 billion annually to care for victims of violence, compared with $10 billion for victims of AIDS (Stolberg 1993).

These data have led to attempts to find ways to "cure" antisocial acts through medical means. A *Los Angeles Times* reporter expressed the hope in the following way: "Could traditional medicine hold clues, even tiny ones, to making streets safe again?" (Stolberg 1993). Various drugs, for example, have been prescribed for people with Huntington disease to control neurotransmitters that appear to cause aggression (see, e.g., Sandyk 1992; Stewart et al. 1987).[43] Dr. Markku Linnoila of the National Institutes of Health found that people with low levels of serotonin are prone to impulsive, violent acts (Stolberg 1993). He is now searching for genes that may cause this imbalance. As the reporter noted, "Finding these genes could help scientists predict who might become violent and give them preventive treatment" (Stolberg 1993). The type of treatment envisioned might be extremely interventionist. After the publication of the findings on MAOA (dubbed the "mean" gene by one journalist), radio talk show hosts suggested sterilizing people who had the gene (Mann 1994, 1689). A writer for *Science Digest* suggested that children who might have a genetic propensity to criminal behavior should be operated on, just as defective cars are recalled and fixed (Taylor 1982).

Some experts have suggested that "half of the prison population is there because their genes predispose them to ADHD (attention deficit hyperactivity disorder)" (Jones 1996, 1).[44] Given the large numbers, it would seem likely that prison officials could make a case for attempting to reduce crime by treating that large group.

Because of our current concern with crime and both political parties' get-tough-on-crime activities, legislatures and state officials have been willing to force offenders to undergo medical treatment to prevent them from committing crimes, even when those interventions have not been proven to be effective and even when the interventions have serious side effects. In 1996 in California, the legislature passed a bill permitting chemical castration of repeat child molesters (Morain and Vanzi 1996).[45] This occurred despite the fact that there is no good evidence that the intervention prevents child molestation, and the drugs have side effects, such as causing the user to grow breasts, gain weight, and suffer from osteoporosis (Kolata 1996).

In 1992, the National Research Council produced a 464-page report, *Understanding and Preventing Violence*, that suggested that new medications could be developed to prevent violence "without undesirable side effects" (Stolberg 1993). Even if such a pie-in-the-sky solution could be obtained, however, it might be discriminatorily applied. "Let's just assume we find a genetic link (to violence)," said Ronald Walters, a political scientist at Howard University, in Washington, D.C. "The question I have always raised is: How will this finding be used? There is a good case, on the basis of history, that it could be used in a racially oppressive way, which is to say you could mount drug programs in inner-city communities based upon this identification of so-called genetic markers" (Stolberg 1993).[46]

There is much evidence that this will be the case, for two reasons. First, stereotypes about race and crime may make it more likely that researchers will look for a gene for aggression or criminality in a minority population—and thus interventions will be applicable only to that population. Along those lines, a long-term study of delinquency followed the children born to 2,958 black mothers (Denno 1989). In Pennsylvania, state police instructed bank employees to take photos of suspicious-looking blacks—thus setting the stage for creation of a criminal profile that applied only to blacks.[47]

Second, our country's criminal laws have long been applied in discriminatory ways. During the time of slavery, slaves were punished for acts that were legal if they were performed by whites (Roberts 1993). After the Emancipation Proclamation, southern legislators passed laws that imprisoned freed slaves on minor offenses (Johnson 1995). Various studies show that even today blacks are treated more harshly in the criminal justice system. Black individuals are more likely to be prosecuted than white individuals, and black individuals receive harsher sentences than whites for similar crimes (Johnson 1995, 636–637).[48] Pregnant white women are slightly more likely to abuse drugs than pregnant black women, but pregnant black women are 9.58 times as likely to be reported for substance abuse during pregnancy.[49] Moreover, offenses that are seen as primarily black are punished more harshly than white offenses—for example, the use of crack cocaine is subject by statute to longer prison sentences than the use of powder cocaine (Johnson 1995, 644). In addition, the stereotype of the violent criminal as a black has fueled erroneous manhunts, such as when, after drowning her children, Susan Smith claimed a black man was responsible (Johnson 1995, 630–631). More generally, surveillance has been used discriminatorily against men of color, to the point where it has been found justifiable to detain black or Hispanic men and search them if they are found in primarily white neighborhoods (Johnson 1995, 655, citing *State v. Dean* 1975 and *State v. Ruiz* 1973).

Even though there is evidence that black people are discriminated against in surveillance activities, arrests, and sentencing, it is often taken for granted that their higher representation in arrests and in prison means they are more violence prone. It is not uncommon, for example, to find statements like the following in newspaper articles: "A disproportionate amount of America's violent crimes (45 percent of murders, rapes and robberies) is committed by black Americans, who make up only 12 percent of the population" (Boseley 1995). This may lead to the disproportionate use of genetic testing and "remedial" interventions in blacks.

Only in rare instances is the differential treatment of blacks and whites seen as sufficiently unjust to be considered a violation of equal protection.[50] For example, even though punishing use of crack cocaine more harshly than use of powder cocaine has not been held to violate the federal constitutional guarantees of equal protection, the Minnesota Supreme Court held that it violates the equal protection clause of the Minnesota constitution (*State v. Russell* 1991).[51]

Surveillance

The state might also decide to keep people with a "crime gene" under surveillance (Green 1973, 571), or keep their profiles on file to be consulted first when a crime is committed.[52] In fact, the law enforcement system might want to take into consideration not just genes for criminal behavior, but genes thought to be associated with precursors to criminal behavior. For example, "[s]tudies of murder, rape, assault, and domestic abuse have reported that alcohol is a factor in the majority of cases" (Coffey 1993, 381). Given enough resources, law enforcement officers may want to keep people with an "alcoholism gene" under surveillance or run their forensic profiles first when trying to find a match to tissue found at a crime scene.

Our society is making increasing use of monitoring and surveillance to deter inappropriate behavior. People are using such tactics in their personal lives. For example, some parents have purchased Drive-right monitors, which keep track of how fast their teenagers drive. Data from the monitor are downloaded into a home computer to show the teen's driving speeds and accelerations (Diamond 1996). Other parents use PDT-90 hair analysis kits to test their children's hair for evidence of drug use (Diamond 1996). Employers monitor employees through such diverse measures as drug tests and electronic counting of key strokes.

State institutions and federal agencies have also adopted a wide range of surveillance and monitoring mechanisms, and in recent years measures that previously would not have been upheld as constitutional have passed muster in the courts.[53] In 1989, for example, the school district in the small logging community of Veronia, Oregon, adopted a policy under which students on sports teams would be required to undergo random urinalysis for drugs. A seventh grader, James Acton, and his parents challenged the policy in court after they refused to consent to the urinalyses and James was barred from sports. His father testified that suspicionless testing "sends a message to children that are trying to be responsible citizens that they have to prove that they're innocent . . . and I think that kind of sets a bad tone for citizenship" (*Veronia School District 47J v. Acton* 1995, 2405).

Even though the Fourth Amendment of the U.S. Constitution had historically protected people against random searches and seizures unless there was individualized suspicion[54] (and urinalysis is considered to be a search) (see, e.g., *Skinner v. Railway Labor Executives' Ass'n* 1989; *National Treasury Employees Union v. Von Raab* 1989), the U.S. Supreme Court in 1995 upheld the random urinalysis policy (*Veronia School District 47J v. Acton* 1995).[55] The Court stated that the "Fourth Amendment does not protect all subjective expectations of privacy, but only those that society recognizes as 'legitimate'" (*Veronia School District 47J v. Acton* 1995, 2391).[56] Legitimacy, however, is an extremely malleable concept. In that case, the Court held that students—especially athletes who undress in front of others—should not expect too much privacy, that urinalyses are not truly intrusive,[57] and that the government had an important interest in deterring a major drug problem.

Random stops of individuals thought to fit criminal profiles of hijackers or drug smugglers have also been upheld as not violating individuals' Fourth Amendment rights (see, e.g., *United States v. Martinez-Fuerte* 1976).[58] The courts have seemed particularly persuaded by the "scientific" nature of the "profiling." One judge referred to the hijacker profiles as "elegant and objective" (*United States v. Lopez* 1971, 1081). He was convinced that research findings had shown that hijackers had characteristics "markedly distinguishing them from the general traveling public" (*United States v. Lopez* 1971, 1082).[59] His analysis of why the standards pass constitutional muster included language that could easily apply to some forms of genetic testing: "Those characteristics selected can be easily observed without exercising judgment. They do not discriminate against any group on the basis of religion, origin, political views, or race. They are precisely designed to select only those who present a high probability of being dangerous. Thus, they violate none of the traditional equal protection standards" (*United States v. Lopez* 1971, 1087, citation omitted).[60]

Nevertheless, certain profiles are administered in racially discriminatory ways. When race is the sole factor used to justify "suspicion" for a search, the action may be seen as unconstitutional under the Fourth Amendment.[61] However, criminal profiles that assess a number of different characteristics, such as profiles to predict who is a drug smuggler, have been upheld even when they are likely to be applied in a discriminatory way.[62]

In the surveillance cases, concern about drugs has been used to justify surveillance policies "based on hunch and whim rather than any reasonable level of suspicion" (*United States v. Taylor* 1992, 590, Martin, J., dissenting). In this era of concern about crime, genetic rationales for surveillance could easily be used, even if they have not been well proven, and even if they discriminate against particular groups.[63]

Preventive Detention

If a gene is identified that is thought to correlate highly with violent behavior—and social and medical means do not appear to prevent the manifestation of violence—then it might be suggested that individuals with the genes be preventively detained so as not to risk harm to others. To the extent that violence is medicalized and seen as a public health problem, this action may be likened to quarantine and justified as a way to protect the public against risk, as was done earlier this century to protect the public against the risk of smallpox or tuberculosis. To some people, the case for isolating people with a gene allegedly linked to violence would be more compelling than quarantining someone with AIDS. A member of the public can protect himself or herself from acquiring AIDS by not having unprotected intercourse, sharing needles, or otherwise engaging in high-risk behaviors. However, a member of the public cannot adequately protect himself or herself from a random violent act.

Normally, confinement would not occur without a prior proven criminal act. U.S. Supreme Court Justices Black and Harlan explained the reason for this requirement: "Evidence of propensity can be considered relatively unreliable and more difficult for a defendant to rebut; the requirement of a specific act thus provides some protection against false charges. Perhaps more fundamental is the difficulty of distinguishing, in the absence of any conduct, between desires of the day-dream variety and fixed intentions that may pose a real threat to society" (*Powell v. Texas* 1968, Black and Harlan, JJ., concurring). Another court noted "our criminal law is based on the theory that we do not condemn people because they are potentially dangerous. We only prosecute illegal acts. Putting a group of potential violators in custody on the grounds that this group contained all or nearly all of the people who would commit crimes in the future would raise most serious constitutional issues" (*United States v. Lopez* 1971, 1100).

However, if "crime" genes were seen as predicting violent behavior, the individual could be civilly committed under the standard of posing "a risk to self or others." Moreover, there may be great leeway in what is considered to be an antisocial act justifying punishment. The study of MAOA deficiency defined the abnormal behavior predicted by the gene to include impulsive aggression, arson, attempted rape, and exhibitionism. It may be that if someone exhibits a nonviolent behavior allegedly associated with a genetic syndrome (such as exhibitionism), courts will be willing to incarcerate the individual on the grounds that this is a prior act that predicts a future violent act, such as attempted rape.

Some Supreme Court justices have viewed incarceration as beneficial in protecting the individual defendant from harm. Justices Black and Harlan, in a case involving public drunkenness, recounted how alcoholics who are jailed are protected from physical danger, such as being run over by a car while intoxicated (*Powell v. Texas* 1968, Black and Harlan, JJ., concurring). The justices pointed out that although jail hardly seems to be "therapeutic" in a traditional sense, there is no generally effective method for curing alcoholics (*Powell v. Texas* 1968, Black and Harlan, JJ., concurring). This sort of logic would justify incarcerating people with a wide range of currently untreatable genetic mutations who might appear in public while disoriented. Justices Black and Harlan also noted that "Apart from the value of jail as a form of treatment, . . . it gets the alcoholics off the street where they may cause harm in a number of ways to a number of people, and isolation of the dangerous has always been considered an important function of the criminal law."

Other Legal Applications

As genetic evidence of antisocial acts becomes increasingly accepted by the courts, it could be used outside of strict criminal prosecutions. One domain in which it might be considered relevant is that of termination of parental rights. Already, in one such case, a judge has mandated that a mother undergo testing for Huntington disease (*Berkeley County Department of Social Services v. David Galley and Kimberly Galley* 1994). State statutes that allow termination of parental rights based on unfitness often specify particular behaviors that are indications of unfitness. These include certain behaviors—such as cruelty, alcoholism, and mental or physical incapacity, sexual promiscuity, and criminal activity (see, e.g., Illinois Revised Statutes 1994)—that are purported to have a genetic basis. Other behaviors, such as moral unfitness, may also be alleged to have a genetic basis.

Parents have been declared unfit when genetic disorders, such as schizophrenia, manifest in ways that cause them to provide inadequate care for their children (*D.W. v. State Department of Human Resources* 1992; *Krystle D. v. Brenda D.* 1994; *David B. v. Lucy B.* 1994). Courts may now want to prevent neglect by terminating rights on the basis of a potential genetic predisposition. Whether a parent could have a child taken from him or her based on the parent having a gene related to antisocial acts would require an analysis similar to the cases in which an individual was deprived of liberty based on such a gene. The U.S. Supreme Court has indicated that a parent's right to the continued custody of his or her children is an "interest far more precious than property rights" (*Lassiter v. Department of Social Services* 1981). To warrant termination, the state must show "a powerful countervailing interest" (*Stanley v. Illinois* 1972).

The Social Implications of the Use of Behavioral
Genetics in the Criminal Justice System

The use of evidence of genetic propensities either to gain liberty (by exculpating defendants) or to curtail liberty (in attempts to prevent antisocial acts) has implications beyond the criminal justice system. It will send a message about the worth of people with certain genotypes and may influence other social uses of behavioral genetics.

Because genetic research is not proceeding at the same pace for all disorders, genetic defenses will be available for some defendants and not others. This may provide an advantage or disadvantage to certain defendants. If a genetic defense exculpates an individual, those whose disorders appear to have a genetic link may be benefited.[64] However, it is more likely in this tough-on-crime era that people who are identified as having "criminal" genes will be stigmatized and treated more harshly. Moreover, unlike the case of genetic testing related to health care, in which disorders that affect powerful majorities are likely to get funded,[65] stereotypes concerning crime may make it more likely that research for genes related to violence will be sought in people of color. Given how easy it is to "see" a genetic link for a complex behavior even when one does not exist,[66] it is likely that minority males will be identified as having genetic propensities to crime and will be disadvantaged as a result.

The use of genetic information by the criminal justice system can stigmatize the relatives of the individuals using those defenses, as well as unrelated third parties who have the same genotype. When Stephen Mobley claimed that a genetic propensity toward violence ran in his family (see Curriden 1994), his father, a multimillionaire businessman, was "embarrassed" by the publicity given to their family history (Verkraik 1995). Such a defense may also stigmatize the ethnic group to which the individual belongs. Consider John Baker, the California lawyer who avoided disbarment by claiming that he was genetically predisposed to alcoholism. That defense was developed by Baker's lawyer *after* Baker mentioned that his father had American Indian blood.[67] Its acceptance in this case may fuel the stereotype that Native Americans are prone to alcoholism.

When the gene at issue is one for a medical condition, people with that condition may be stigmatized as well. Philip Cohen, a spokesman for the Huntington's Disease Society of America, raised concern that Caldwell's acquittal of her son's murder might stigmatize other people who have Huntington disease as being violent (AP 1994).[68] I saw evidence of this among the students in the class I was teaching on genetics and the law during the semester in which the Caldwell acquittal was rendered. If Caldwell's disease made her uncontrollably prone to violence, asserted my students, it would seem to follow that people would have a duty to learn whether they had the gene and that the people with the gene and their physicians would have a duty to warn relatives and other third parties that these people presented a genetic risk of violence.[69]

The acceptance of genetic predictions of antisocial behavior in the criminal context might lead to other social uses of the tests. At a Ciba Foundation Symposium in England, Dr. David Goldman of the U.S. National Institutes of Health said that prenatal information about a fetus's predisposition to antisocial behavior should be given to families, with a decision about whether to abort made privately (Moore 1995). The Dutch family in which an alleged link was found between a gene for MAOA deficiency and aggression is now faced with the question of whether they should use the test for prenatal screening (Highfield 1995).

Conclusion

It is unlikely that geneticists will locate a gene, or even a set of genes, that invariably predisposes an individual to antisocial acts. However, based on small studies of individual families, some researchers may claim that such genes exist. Such researchers—as well as clinical geneticists—may be willing to go into court and testify, as happened in the XYY cases, that a particular genetic profile "caused" a person to commit a crime. This genetic determinism will be appealing to judges and other policymakers, who do not feel they have the resources to deal with the complex social factors that seem somehow connected to criminal behavior (for example, the low education and self-esteem of people who commit crimes, the fact that the majority of people on Death Row have been in foster care, and so forth). Moreover, the genes-equal-crimes equation will strike a chord with society at large which, in this blame-the-victim era, finds comfort in explanations that are internal to the individual, thus eliminating society's responsibility to attempt to remedy the situation.

The politics of difference provide the backdrop against which the information about behavioral genetics will be incorporated into criminal justice practices. If genes are thought to predispose to antisocial acts, people may wish to take a variety of measures to protect themselves against individuals with "criminal" genes. Society may feel safer if those "others" are identified, kept under surveillance, and "treated." There is ample reason to believe that these measures, like existing criminal justice measures, will be implemented in a way that continues to discriminate against men and women of color.

Acknowledgments

This work was supported by a grant from the National Center for Human Genome Research, National Institutes of Health, R01-HG01277-01.

Notes

1. One of the researchers acknowledged the limitations as follows: "What we have reported is a single observation. . . . If the next family with MAOA deficiency is completely normal, that gives a whole set of new questions" (Boseley 1995).

2. The court refused to authorize testing for MAOA deficiency, saying "the theory of genetic connection is not at a level of scientific acceptance that would justify its admission" (Curriden 1994). Mobley was convicted and sentenced to death.

3. "In criminal law, for example, whether one takes a philosophic or economic approach, some concept of responsibility is essential to most forms of culpability" (Dreyfuss and Nelkin 1992).

4. In California, in the early 1980s, there were 12 prisons housing about 20,000 inmates. Now there are at least 32 prisons with over 140,000 inmates (Editorial [1996]. See also Opinion (1996).

5. In some instances, the conditions in these prisons are so extreme that they have been found to be unconstitutional. A federal district court found unconstitutional conditions in the maximum security housing unit at Pelican Bay prison in California (Bendavid and Mintz 1996). The court ruled that the conditions were cruel and unusual and caused "senseless suffering and sometimes wretched misery" (Raine 1996). The U.S. Department of Justice threatened to sue state officials in Maryland over conditions at its "Supermax" prison, formally known as the Maryland Correctional Adjustment Center (Shatzkin 1996).

6. This is part of an age-old search for biological correlates of criminality. "In the past, criminality has been associated with everything from race to physical features and body structure" (Coffey 1993, 353–354, footnotes omitted).

7. Her optimism about the ease with which the genetic underpinnings of behavior will be found is not supported by scientific evidence. See note 66.

8. Recent research claims to have found a genetic disposition for pathological gambling (Gregory 1996).

9. "With the new genetics, it is becoming easier to blame all bad conduct on DNA. Acts once thought of as the result of poor upbringing are more and more ascribed to inborn weakness" (Jones 1996).

10. *Yukl v. New York*, 83 Misc. 2d 364, 372 N.Y.S. 2d 313, 320 (1997) discusses the Australian case.

11. "To identify a 'criminal gene' seems as primitive as Lombroso's nineteenth-century notion of dividing up the swindlers from murderers on the basis of facial characteristics. Yet why does this kind of genetic reductionism hold such sway? Possibly because so few of us really understand much about neurotransmitters, the amygdala, and the controversial claim that there is a link between 'a point mutation in the structural gene monoamine oxidase inhibitor' and abnormal behavior.

"Any geneticist worth his or her salt might care to locate precisely the gene which causes a predisposition to abandoning all our critical faculties so that we do indeed become blinded by science. Social scientists on the other hand could undertake a study which would show us who is funding this sort of research and why" (Moore 1995).

12. See also Nelkin and Lindee (1996). Glenda Sue Caldwell, accused of murdering her son, was found not guilty by reason of insanity due to her Huntington disease. She said "I always knew that something was wrong with me. I was not responsible for what I did. I'm a good person" (*Bergen Record* 1994).

13. In *Caldwell v. State* (1987), for example, the defendant raised a defense related to stress from her marital separation.

14. See, e.g., *People v. Newton* (1970), where the court reversed Newton's conviction for killing a police officer because the judge failed to give the jury an exculpatory instruction based on evidence that Newton fired his gun in an involuntary reflex shock condition after he had been shot in the stomach. See also *Wise v. Florida* (1991).

15. This is relevant not only to the question of whether the individual is seen as being guilty of the crime but also whether the individual can be executed. *Ford v. Wainwright* (1986) holds that an insane individual may not be executed.

16. This is what happened to a woman with the Huntington disease mutation in the *Caldwell* case, discussed later. A finding of insanity may be no great bargain for the defendant, however, since he or she may be committed to a mental health facility. Historically, in England such a verdict "resulted in commitment to a hospital during the king's or queen's pleasure and it so seldom pleased the monarch to do anything about the matter that the normal result was hospitalization for life, for which reason the plea was used only as a last resort" (Perkins and Boyce 1982, 990, footnote omitted). Now, however, such institutionalizations are subject to periodic review. Since an individual's genetic constitution is generally immutable, however, it may be difficult for an individual who has used a genetic defense to prove that he or

she should be released, unless a new treatment or gene therapy becomes available to significantly change his or her behavior.

17. A variety of individuals raising genetic defenses have been found "guilty but mentally ill." This was the first trial outcome in *Caldwell v. State* (1987). Likewise, the defendants in *Scammahorn v. State* (1987) and in *Tenney v. State* (1985) were found guilty but mentally ill. In all three instances, the defendants had Huntington disease.

18. Deborah Denno argues that genetic defenses should not be allowed for exculpation, except in rare instances in which the genetic condition causes insanity for that particular defendant. She suggests instead that they be used at the sentencing stage, not to reduce the length of sentence, but to determine the type of facility in which the convicted defendant should be institutionalized (Denno 1988, 617).

19. Coffey notes that "theoretically, society would gain little satisfaction in seeking retribution against one who is neither responsible for, nor capable of changing, his physical constitution. Under such circumstances, retribution would be, in effect, exacting vengeance for a birth defect" (Coffey 1993, 392–393). Society may, however, be more coldhearted than Coffey asserts. In other areas, society has been willing to "blame the victim."

20. Revenge seems to be a primary motive behind the "three strikes" law.

21. "Although an individual, through no fault of her own, may be born with an immutable predisposition to behavior that society has deemed unacceptable, in some cases the normative ends—for example, removing a potentially dangerous offender from the street—may justify the morally debatable means" (Coffey 1993, 398).

22. The fact that policymakers have "written off" people convicted of a crime is evident by recent policy measures, including the dismantling of education programs geared toward prisoners and the conversion of classrooms in prisons into additional dormitory space. A Wisconsin state lawmaker, Rob G. Kreibich, introduced a bill that prohibited state prisoners from receiving college tuition grants, thus, in his words "ending an outrageous waste of state tax dollars" (Kreibich 1996). Such an approach is enormously shortsighted, though. Given that 95 percent of prisoners are ultimately released, it would seem better for society at large if they were sufficiently well educated to have a better chance of getting a job.

23. In *Powell v. Texas* (1968, 531), the U.S. Supreme Court felt that bans on public drunkenness would have a deterrent effect by "reinforc[ing] this cultural taboo [against appearing drunk in public] just as we presume it serves to reinforce other, stronger feelings against murder, rape, theft, and other forms of antisocial conduct."

24. The Court did indicate that "a State might determine that the general health and welfare require that the victims of these and other human afflictions be dealt with by compulsory treatment, involving quarantine, confinement, or sequestration."

25. Justice Douglas noted that the "impact that an addict has on a community

causes alarm and often leads to punitive measures. Those measures are justified when they relate to acts of transgression. But I do not see how under our system being an addict can be punished as a crime."

26. The Court said it "has never held that anything in the Constitution requires that penal sanctions be designed solely to achieve therapeutic or rehabilitative effects, and it can hardly be said with assurance that incarceration serves such purposes any better for the general run of criminals that it does for public drunks."

27. The Court also indicated that "a State might choose to attack the evils of narcotics traffic on broader fronts also—through public health education, for example, or by efforts to ameliorate the economic and social considerations under which those evils might be thought to flourish." Today, however, such economic and social responses are far less likely to be undertaken.

28. The challenge that genetics poses for criminal law may not be as great as Dan Brock (1992) suggests, since historically the law has not required evidence of free will, but presumed it. As Herbert Packer noted three decades ago, "Neither philosophic concepts nor psychological realities are actually at issue in the criminal law. The idea of free will in relation to conduct is not, in the legal system, a statement of fact, but rather a value preference having very little to do with the metaphysics of determinism and free will. . . . Very simply, the law treats man's conduct as autonomous and willed, not because it is, but because it is desirable to proceed as if it were" (Packer 1968, 74–75).

29. In this case, the defendant was charged with kidnapping, forcible rape, and assault with intent to commit murder. The court sent him to Atascadero State Hospital for study. There, "appellant was discovered to possess cells with an extra male or Y chromosome" (*People v. Tanner* 1970, 588). No mention is made in the decision about why the state hospital was testing its patients' chromosomes, or even if the defendant had been asked for consent prior to the test.

At trial, two geneticists testified that 47 XYY individuals exhibit aggressive behavior as a causal result of this chromosomal abnormality (*People v. Tanner* 1970, 658–659). The court, however, held that "the studies of the '47 XYY individuals' undertaken to this time are few, they are rudimentary in scope, and their results are at best inconclusive" (*People v. Tanner* 1970, 659). The court ruled that the studies did not indicate that all XYY individuals are involuntarily aggressive, nor did the experts prove whether the defendant's aggressive behavior resulted from his chromosomal abnormality (*People v. Tanner* 1970, 600–601).

30. In that case, the defendant's expert witness was geneticist Cecil Jacobson, a medical professor at George Washington University (who, twenty years later himself ran afoul of the law when, as director of an infertility clinic, he used his own sperm to inseminate patients). Dr. Jacobson "told of approximately 40 published reports indicating that persons possessed of an extra Y chromosome tended to be very tall,

with limbs disproportionate to their body; that such persons had marked antisocial, aggressive and schizoid relations and were in continual conflict with the law." His testimony indicated that the defendant had a "propensity" toward the commission of crime. Nevertheless, Jacobson conceded that persons with the extra Y chromosome differ among themselves. Also, since Jacobson was not a psychiatrist, he felt he was not competent to answer whether the defendant had substantial capacity to appreciate the consequences of his actions. In contrast, the state's six psychiatric witnesses indicated that the defendant was not insane. The trial judge consequently decided not to allow an insanity defense. The jury found the defendant guilty of robbery with a deadly weapon, which was upheld on appeal, and he was sentenced to eighteen years in prison. Nevertheless, if the defendant had procured his own psychiatric witness, he might have prevailed because Jacobson's testimony made it seem as if there was no doubt that he had a criminal gene.

31. The two cases are compared in Dreyfuss and Nelkin (1992, 328–331).

32. Such was the advice in a November 29, 1994 philanthropy journal.

33. In *Knight v. Texas* (1975), overruled on other grounds, *Johnson v. State* (1977), the defendant made a motion (which was denied) requesting "at least $1,000 be allowed for medical examination and tests" to determine if he had the XYY chromosomal complement. Some expert testimony must be accessible to indigent defendants. The U.S. Supreme Court has held that it is an unconstitutional deprivation of due process under the Fourth Amendment for a state not to provide access to a psychiatrist for an indigent defendant who has made a preliminary showing that his sanity will be at issue in the case (*Ake v. Oklahoma* 1985).

The court included a quotation from Goldstein and Lane, in *Goldstein Trial Technique* (1969) that suggests that the state's duty to pay for experts might go beyond paying for psychiatrists: "Modern civilization, with its complexities of business, science, and the professions, has made expert and opinion evidence a necessity. This is true whether the subject matters are beyond the general knowledge of the average juror" (Goldstein and Lane 1969, 82).

34. The judge considered three statutory aggravating circumstances: murder committed while in the commission of a rape; murder committed while in the commission of kidnapping; and murder committed during armed robbery. However, the judge also considered mitigating circumstances, including that Roach was a minor, mentally retarded, and his capacity to appreciate the criminality of his conduct or to conform his conduct to the requirements of the law was substantially impaired (*Roach v. Martin* 1985, 1468).

35. Harold Green notes that society might also try to restrict marriages when the couple might produce a child with a genetic propensity to antisocial acts, or abortion might be made mandatory if the condition were diagnosed in a fetus (Green 1973, 571).

36. In 1994, Congress passed a law granting an average of $8 million per year for five years to facilitate states' establishment of DNA banks. 42 U.S.C. § 13701 (1996).

37. See, for example, *Jones v. Murray* (1992). However, in that case, Judge Murnaghan, concurring and dissenting, argued that DNA testing of nonviolent felons is unconstitutional (*Jones v. Murray* 1992, 313).

38. A Virginia statute prohibits unauthorized dissemination of information from the forensic DNA data banks, but there is no guidance as to what is considered unauthorized use (Virginia Code Ann. 1995).

39. In fact, once a gene is uncovered that purports to predispose individuals to antisocial acts, law enforcement officials may feel *obligated* to act on it. One court has noted that if a passenger about to board a plane fits the hijacker profile, "[a] United States Marshal would be imprudent were he to refuse to heed the warning given to him by the system" (*United States v. Lopez* 1971, 1097).

40. It should be noted, too, that this was not a study of *genetic* predisposition to crime. Rather, the factors that correlated with a high degree of aggression in these men's lives were environmental—harsh punishment as children, watching violent television shows as children, and neglect or rejection as children (Hilts 1983).

41. In addition, a few states protect the privacy of genetic information, although generally these laws apply only to genetic information obtained through DNA analysis. For example, a Florida law states that DNA analysis results "are the exclusive property of the person tested, are confidential, and may not be disclosed without the consent of the person tested" (Florida Stat. Ann. 1995).

42. Such an approach has allowed CDC to enhance its budget. President Clinton endorsed a special CDC line item to fund violence prevention programs (Stolberg 1993, II).

43. "Treatment" might also consist of *avoiding* certain medications. For example, amantadine given for treatment of influenza caused a marked increase in irritability and aggressiveness in two patients with Huntington disease (Stewart 1987).

44. Jones notes, "If this is true, prisons are as much institutions for the genetically unlucky as places of punishment."

45. In contrast, legislators in the Netherlands rejected such an approach (ANP English news bulletin 1996).

46. For examples of improper medical experimentation on black individuals, see Washington (1994).

47. This action was held to create a cause of action under the Civil Rights Act on behalf of a black who was photographed. "The photography program initiated by the state policy is a form of criminal investigation directed against the plaintiff because of his race" (*Hall v. Pennsylvania State Police* 1978).

48. Prosecutors in Georgia sought the death penalty in 70 percent of cases involving black defendants and white victims, and 32 percent of cases involving white defendants and black victims (*McCleskey v. Kemp* 1987, discussing a study by Profes-

sors David C. Baldus, Charles Pulaski and George Woodworth). The study also found that the death penalty was assessed in 22 percent of the cases involving black defendants and white victims, as opposed to 3 percent of cases involving white defendants and black victims (*McCleskey v. Kemp* 1987, 286).

49. This was the finding of a Florida study of 715 women (Moss 1990, 294, citation omitted). Other surveys of prosecutions of pregnant women indicate that "despite evidence that illegal drug use is the same across race and class lines, women of color, and poor women are the ones who are being prosecuted" (Paltrow 1992, iii–iv, citing Chasnoff et al. 1990; Kolata 1990, 13; Roberts 1991). Overall, "while blacks account for only 12% of our nations' drug users, between 80% and 90% of those arrested for any drug offense are young black men" (Johnson 1995, 641).

50. The Fourteenth Amendment to the U.S. Constitution provides that no state shall "deny to any person within its jurisdiction the equal protection of the laws." In addition, violations of equal protection are violations of due process under the Fifth Amendment (*Bolling v. Sharpe* 1954).

51. In 1988, 96.6 percent of the people charged with possession of crack were black. Of those charged with powder cocaine, 79.6 percent were white (*State v. Russell* 1991, 887 n.1).

52. For an illuminating novel based on this premise, see Kerr (1992).

53. See, e.g., *United States v. Knotts* (1983) (police use of an electronic tracking instrument on a car does not violate the Fourth Amendment). For a discussion of the privacy implications of the use of such devices, see McAdams (1985).

54. *Veronia School District 47J v. Acton* (1995) (O'Connor, Stevens, and Souter, JJ., dissenting). The dissenting Justices, citing LaFave 1987, pointed out that "it remains the law that the police cannot, say, subject to drug testing every person entering or leaving a certain drug-ridden neighborhood in order to find evidence of crime.... And this is true even though it is hard to think of a more compelling governmental interest than the need to fight the scourge of drugs on our streets and in our neighborhoods" (LaFave 1987, 2400). Another judge has noted that the use of the antihijacking profile results in finding a weapon on 6 percent of the individuals being frisked (*United States v. Lopez* 1971). "Mere statistical information such as that generated in this case does not, by itself, justify 'frisks.' If, for example, reliable statistics were available that in a given community one person in fifteen (six percent) regularly carried concealed weapons [the] police would not be justified in arbitrarily stopping and frisking anyone on the street. Such harassment by police without more objective evidence of criminal activity or a legitimate investigative purpose is proscribed by the Fourth Amendment" (*United States v. Lopez* 1971, 1097–1098, citations omitted).

55. The court noted that its holding was based in part on the fact that a school is the guardian of the children entrusted to its care (*Veronia School District 47J v. Acton* 1995, 2396).

56. The Court did indicate that some privacy concerns might be relevant. "In this

regard it is significant that the tests at issue here look only for drugs, and not whether the student is, for example, epileptic, pregnant, or diabetic" (*Veronia School District 47J v. Acton* 1995, 2393).

57. This perception has not historically been the case. "In our culture the excretory functions are shielded by more or less absolute privacy" (Fried 1968).

58. *United States v. Martinez-Fuerte* (1976) (upholding Border Patrol checkpoint stops and further detention of some individuals for questioning absent individualized suspicion). The dissenting justices noted the discriminatory effect of such a policy, "Every American citizen of Mexican ancestry and every Mexican alien lawfully in this country must know after today's decision that he travels the fixed checkpoint highways at the risk of not only being subjected to a stop, but also to detention and interrogation both prolonged and to an extent far more [than] for non-Mexican appearing motorists" (*United States v. Martinez-Fuerte* 1976, 572, Brennan and Marshall, JJ., dissenting). They noted further that "even if good faith is assumed, the affront to the dignity of American citizens of Mexican ancestry and Mexican aliens lawfully within the country is in no way diminished" (*United States v. Martinez-Fuerte* 1976, 573, n.4).

59. In fact, he held an *in camera* hearing from which he excluded the defendant on the grounds that "were even one characteristic of the 'profile' generally revealed, the system could be seriously undermined by hijackers fabricating an acceptable profile" (*United States v. Lopez* 1971, 1086).

60. The court approved of the use of the profile, but held that it was improperly administered in this case, in which airline employees added an ethnic component as well (*United States v. Lopez* 1971, 1101). The court noted, however, "We reach this conclusion recognizing that the system used is disquieting. Employing a combination of psychological, sociological, and physical sciences to screen, inspect and categorize unsuspecting citizens raises visions of abuse in our increasingly technological society. Proposals based upon statistical research designed to predict who might commit crimes and giving them the special attention of law enforcement officials is particularly disturbing" (*United States v. Lopez* 1971, 1100).

61. *United States v. Beck* (1979), in which a police search of a car was held to be improper. The court said, "There is nothing inherently suspicious about two black men sitting in a parked car, with or without the engine running, on a street in a black neighborhood on a midsummer afternoon" (*United States v. Beck* 1979, 729).

62. Some of the factors asserted by law enforcement officials to raise suspicion that someone is a drug smuggler are so broad as to invite discriminatory application. In one case, Pennsylvania state troopers stopped a man for speeding and then detained him for two and a half hours as a suspected drug smuggler because he seemed nervous; he asked to go to the bathroom; his car had a lot of miles on it; he had fast-food wrappers and vegetable matter in the car; his car had license plates from

Florida, a known drug center; he was traveling on a highway to Harrisburg, allegedly a regional drug trade center; the car had a car phone antenna; and the car was a mid-sized blue Honda. The troopers argued "that mid to full size cars and cars which are average looking or common and which easily blend in with traffic are frequently used to transport drugs" (*Karnes v. Skrutski* 1995). The trial court had held that these reasons were sufficient to justify the search, but the appellate court pointed out that many innocent people would meet this profile (*Karnes v. Skrutski* 1995, 495). In addition, it pointed out the absurdity of arguing that having an average car raises suspicion. "Were we to accept this argument, we would be granting permission to conduct investigatory stops of people deemed 'suspiciously normal.' The Fourth Amendment forbids granting such permission" (*Karnes v. Skrutski* 1995, 495). The appellate court remanded the case for a jury determination of reasonable suspicion, opening up the possibility of the plaintiff getting monetary damages for violation of his Fourth Amendment rights.

In another case, Eddie Louis Taylor was the only African American in the initial group of deplaning passengers in Memphis, on a flight from Miami. Three plain-clothes officers from the Memphis police department followed him as a potential drug smuggler since he was agitated, poorly attired, had no checked luggage, and carried a new bag. They claimed his race was not an issue. The district court, upheld by the appellate court, found that detention of Taylor once he was outside the airport, and the search of his bags, which revealed contraband, was "consensual" and thus not in violation of the Fourth Amendment since "a reasonable individual in Taylor's position would have felt free to ignore the officers' invitation to engage in a conversation, and proceed on his way. In this context it is of no consequence that [Police Officer] Eldridge testified that he would have pursued Taylor if he had fled" (*United States v. Taylor* 1992). It seems patently absurd to assume that a black man would feel free to walk away from white law enforcement officials in the South. One only need to remember the Rodney King tape or the incident in which baseball Hall of Famer Joe Morgan was accosted by state agents in Los Angeles International Airport while making a phone call and, when he attempted to identify himself, was thrown to the floor and handcuffed before a crowd of onlookers (*United States v. Taylor* 1992, 583, dissenting opinion).

The dissenting Judge Keith, joined by judges Merritt, Martin, and Jones, pointed out that 75 percent of those questioned in these "consensual" stops are black and argued that the assumption that 75 percent of drug smugglers are black is "impermissible" (*United States v. Taylor* 1992, 581, Keith, Merritt, Martin and Jones, JJ., dissenting). "If our 'right of locomotion,' 'right to be left alone,' or simply our right to be free from capricious and arbitrary government interference in public places is to mean anything, then this race-based practice must stop" (*United States v. Taylor* 1992, 581–582). Judge Martin, in his own separate dissent, underscored that it was simply impermissible, even under the weakened and eroded state of the Fourth Amendment, to justify stopping Taylor just because of the appearance of his clothes, his travel from Miami, and the fact that he was black. Judge Martin pointed out he, too, is sometimes agitated when he flies, but faces little chance of being stopped by the police. "Perhaps it is my dress and manner; I believe it is these factors combined with the fact that I am white" (*United States v. Taylor* 1992, 590, Martin, J., dissenting).

63. Use of criminal profiles was upheld in *United States v. Mendenhall* (1980). For a criticism of the practice, owing to its discriminatory impact on black males, see Johnson (1995).

64. "Some actors may escape punishment while others are convicted, not because of relative guilt, but because members of the former group suffer from problems that are better understood by the medical community" (Dreyfuss and Nelkin 1992, 329–330).

65. For many decades, NIH-funded research focused almost exclusively on white male patients (Dresser 1992; Mastroianni et al. 1994). Even today, diseases that have large, vocal constituencies tend to receive disproportionate funding.

66. Some of the country's more respected genetic researchers have published data identifying genetic links for certain complex behaviors, only to find later that such links did not hold up. For a discussion of the numerous failures to replicate researchers' genetic linkage of common neuropsychiatric disorders (such as schizophrenia, manic-depressive disorder, and Alzheimer disease), see Risch (1990). Risch points out that "there are fundamental differences between the rare, Mendelian disorders and the common 'complex' familial disorders, both in terms of conceptualization and approaches to analysis, that need to be addressed before significant progress can be made in understanding the 'complex' diseases" (Risch 1990, 4). See also Marshall (1994).

67. In describing this sequence of events, Professor Steven Jones notes, "that race's drink problem is well documented" (Jones 1996, 1).

68. In a similar vein, some commentators argue that the postpartum psychosis defense, used successfully in England to obtain "not guilty by reason of insanity" verdicts, might be stigmatizing to women (Holtzman 1986).

69. The students were obviously influenced by *Tarasoff v. Regents of the University of California*, 131 Cal. Rptr. 14, 551 P.2d 334 (1976), in which a psychiatrist was held to have a duty to warn a violent patient's intended victim.

References

Agence France Presse. 1996. Swedish appeals court acquits mother of euthanasia charges. Agence France Presse (March 27).

Ake v. Oklahoma. 1985. 470 U.S. 68, 74 (1985).

Andrews, L., ed. 1985. *State Laws and Regulations Regarding Newborn Screening.* Chicago: American Bar Foundation.

Andrews, L. 1995. Genetic privacy: From the laboratory to the legislature. *Gen. Res.* 5 (Oct.): 209–213.

Andrews, L. 1996. Prenatal screening and the culture of motherhood. *Hastings Law J.* 47: 967.

ANP English news bulletin. 1996. Sorgdrager, MP, reject chemical castration for sex offenders. *Stichting Algemeen Nederlands Persbureau* (Sept. 3) (LEXIS NEWS file).

AP (Associated Press). 1994. Disease cited in murder acquittal. *Cleveland Plain Dealer* (Sept. 29): 6A.

Baker v. State Bar of California. 1989. 781 P.2d 1344, 1353 (Cal. 1989).

Bendavid, N., and H. Mintz. 1996. Judges' authority in prison cases thrown in doubt. *Recorder* (May 6): 1.

Bergen Record. 1994. Blaming illness, woman cleared of killing son (Sept. 19): A15.

Berkeley County Department of Social Services v. David Galley and Kimberly Galley. 1994. 92-DR-08-2699 (Apr. 19, 1994) (ruling of the court).

Bolling v. Sharpe. 1954. 347 U.S. 497 (1954).

Boseley, S. 1995. Second front: Genes in the dock. *Guardian* (Mar. 13): T2.

Brock, D. 1992. The Human Genome Project and human identity. *Houston Law Rev.* 29: 7.

Brunner, H. G., M. Nelen, X. O. Breakefield, et al. 1993. Abnormal behavior associated with a point mutation in the structural gene for monoamine oxidase A. *Science* 262: 578 (Oct. 22).

Brusca, A. D. 1990. Note, post-partum psychosis: A way out for murderous moms? *Hofstra Law Rev.* 18: 1133.

Burke, K. J. 1969. The "XYY syndrome": Genetics, behavior and the law. *University of Denver Law J.* 46: 261.

Caldwell v. State. 1987. 257 Ga. 10, 354 S.E.2d 124 (Ga. 1987).

Carter v. State. 1962. 376 P.2d 351 (Oklahoma Criminal App. 1962).

Chadwin, D. 1996. The DNA war: How two marines fought the military's genetic roundup. *Village Voice* 23 (May 14).

Chasnoff, I. J., H. J. Landress, and M. E. Barrett, 1990. Illicit drug and alcohol use during pregnancy. *N. Engl. J. Med.* 322 (April 26): 1202.

Coffey, M. P. 1993. The genetic defense: Excuse or explanation? *William and Mary Law Rev.* 35: 353–399.

Colorado Statutes Annotated. 1994. §10-3-1104.7(1)(a) and (3)(a) (West 1994).

Curriden, M. 1994. Guilt by heredity? His lawyers say it's in the killer's genes. *Nat. Law J.* A12 (Nov. 7).

D.W. v. State Department of Human Resources. 1992. 595 So.2d 502 (Ala. Civ. App. 1992).

Daubert v. Merrill Dow Pharmaceuticals. 1993. 509 U.S. 579, 590 (1993).

David B. v. Lucy B. 1994. No. A-93-873, 1994 Neb. App. LEXIS 187 (Neb. Ct. App. June 21, 1994).

Denno, D. W. 1988. Human biology and criminal responsibility: Free will or free ride? *University of Pennsylvania Law Rev.* 137: 615–671.

Denno, D. W. 1989. *Biology and Violence: From Birth to Adulthood.* Cambridge, United Kingdom: Cambridge University Press.

Diamond, D. 1996. Keeping tabs on teens. *USA Weekend* (Aug. 30–Sept. 1): 4–5.

Dresser, R. 1992. Wanted: Single white male for medical research. *Hastings Cent. Rep.* 22 (Jan.–Feb.): 24–29.

Dreyfuss, R., and D. Nelkin 1992. The jurisprudence of genetics. *Vanderbilt Law Rev.* 25: 313.

Editorial. 1996. Proposal to improve state's prison industry. *San Francisco Chronicle* (May 26): 8/Z1.

Florida Statutes Annotated. 1995. §760.40(2)(a) (West Supp. 1995).

Ford v. Wainwright. 1986. 477 U.S. 399 (1986).

Freyne, A., and A. O'Connor. 1992. XYY Genotype and crime: Two cases. *Med. Sci. Law* 32: 261.

Fried, C. 1968. Privacy. *Yale Law J.* 77: 475, 487.

Goldstein, I., and R. F. Lane. 1969. *Goldstein Trial Technique,* vol. 2. §14.01 (2d ed.).

Green, H. P. 1973. Genetic technology: Law and policy for the brave new world. *Indiana Law J.* 48: 571.

Gregory, T. 1996. Researcher's theory criticized: Doctor proposes genetic link to gambling. *Chicago Tribune* (Sept. 4): sec. 2, p. 8.

Hall v. Pennsylvania State Police. 1978. 570 F.2d 86 (3d Cir. 1978).

Hart, H. L. 1968. Legal responsibility and excuses. *Punishment and Responsibility* 28: 44.

Herrnstein, R. J., and C. Murray. 1994. *The Bell Curve: Intelligence and Class Structure in American Life.* New York: Free Press.

Hibbert, M. 1998. State DNA banks: Law enforcement's greatest surveillance tool? (unpublished manuscript on file with the author).

Highfield, R. 1995. Scientists can test foetus for violent gene: Discovery may affect U.S. murder trials. *Daily Telegraph* (Feb. 14): 4.

Hilts, P. J. 1983. 8-Year-old bully apt to remain that way. *Washington Post* (Aug. 27): A2.

Holtzman, E. 1986. Premenstrual symptoms: No legal defense. *St. John's Law Rev.* 60: 712.

Illinois Revised Statutes. 1994. ch. 705 para. /1 et seq. (1994).

In re Ewaniszyk. 1990. 788 P.2d 690 (Cal. Ct. App. 1990).

Jacobs, P. A., M. Bruton, M. M. Melville, et al. 1965. Aggressive behavior, mental subnormality, and the XYY male. *Nature* 1208: 351.

Jaroff, L. 1996. Keys in the kingdom. *Time* 24–29 (Fall).

Johnson v. State. 1977. 548 S.W.2d 685 (Tex. Crim. App. 1977).

Johnson, E. L. 1995. "A menace to society": The use of criminal profiles and its effect on black males. *Howard Law J.* 38: 629–664, 635.

Jones v. Murray. 1992. 962 F.2d 302 (4th Cir.), *cert. denied*, 506 U.S. 977.

Jones, S. 1996. The criminal gene. *Daily Telegraph* (Apr. 27): 1.

Kaplan, J., R. Weisberg, and G. Binder. 1996. *Criminal Law: Cases and Materials*, 3d ed., 746. Boston: Little, Brown.

Karnes v. Skrutski. 1995. 62 F.3d 485, 495 (3rd Cir. 1995).

Kerr, P. 1993. *A Philosophical Investigation.* New York: Farrar, Strauss, and Giroux.

Knight v. Texas. 1975. 538 S.W.2d 101, 106 (1975).

Kolata, G. 1990. Racial bias seen on pregnant addicts. *New York Times* (July 20): 13.

Kolata, G. 1995. Gene test poses dilemma for Alzheimer's experts. *International Herald Tribune* (Oct. 26).

Kolata, G. 1996. The many myths about sex offenders. *New York Times* (September 1) Sect. 4, p. 10, col. 1.

Kreibich, R. G. 1996. Hard time or play time: Putting an end to prison perks punishes prisoners and saves money. *Milwaukee Journal Sentinel* (Mar. 17): 1.

Krent, H. J. 1995. Of diaries and data banks: Use regulations under the Fourth Amendment. *Texas Law Rev.* 74: 49–100.

Krystle D. v. Brenda B. 37 Cal. Rptr. 2d 132 (Ct. App. 1994).

LaFave, W. 1987. *Search and Seizure*, vol. 3. §9.5(b), pp. 551–553 (2d ed. 1987).

Lassiter v. Department of Social Services. 1981. 452 U.S. 18, 27 (1981).

Levine, A. M. 1998. Denying the settled insanity defense: Another necessary step in dealing with drugs and alcohol abuse. *Boston University Law Rev.* 78: 75, 80.

Lynch, L. 1996. "Three strikes" and chain gangs struck down in California. Inter Press Service (June 26). (LEXIS, NEWS database).

McAdams, R. H. 1985. Tying privacy in *Knotts:* Beeper monitoring and collective Fourth Amendment rights. *Virginia Law Rev.* 71: 297.

McCleskey v. Kemp. 1987. 481 U.S. 279, 287 (1987).

McEwen, J. E., and P. R. Reilly. 1994a. A review of state legislation on DNA forensic data banking. *Am. J. Hum. Genet.* 54: 941–958.

McEwen, J. E., and P. R. Reilly. 1994b. Stored Guthrie cards as DNA "Banks." *Am. J. Hum. Genet.* 55: 196–200.

Mann, C. C. 1994. Behavioral genetics in transition. *Science* 264: 1686–1689.

Marshall, E. 1994. Highs and lows on the research roller coaster. *Science* 264: 1693–1695.

Mastroianni, A. C., R. Faden, and D. Federman, eds. 1994. *Women and Health Research: Ethical and Legal Issues of Including Women in Clinical Studies.* Washington, D.C.: National Academy Press.

Millard v. State. 1970. 261 A.2d 227 (Md. 1970).

Model Penal Code. 1995. §4.01.

Model Penal Code. 1995. §2.01(2).

Moore, S. 1995. Genetic scientists lost in inner space. *Guardian* (Feb. 16): T5.

Morain, D., and M. Vanzi. 1996. Senate OKs access to sex offenders database. *Los Angeles Times* (Sept. 1): A3.

Moss, K. 1990. Substance abuse during pregnancy. *Harvard Women's Law J.* 13: 278–299.

Nacheman, A. 1995. Violent gene could save U.S. killer from electric chair. Agence France Presse (February 17) (LEXIS, NEWS file).

National Treasury Employees Union v. Von Raab. 1989. 489 U.S. 656, 665 (1989).

Nelkin, D., and M. S. Lindee. 1995. *The DNA Mystique: The Gene as a Cultural Icon*, 145. New York: Freeman.

Nelkin, D., and M. S. Lindee. 1996. 'Genes made me do it': The appeal of biological explanations. *Politics Life Sci.* 15 (Mar.): 95–97.

Opinion. 1996. California's packed prisons pose prickly problems. *San Diego Union-Tribune* (May 8): B-5.

Packer, H. 1968. *The Limits of Criminal Sanction*, 74–75. Stanford, Calif.: Stanford University Press.

Paltrow, L. M. 1992. Reproductive Freedom Project, American Civil Liberties Union Foundation. *Criminal Prosecutions against Pregnant Women: National Update and Overview: April 1992*, iii–iv.

People v. Decina. 1956. 138 N.E.2d 799 (N.Y. 1956).

People v. Newton. 1970. 8 Cal. App. 3d 359 (1970).

People v. Tanner. 1970. 91 Cal. Rptr. 656, 658 n.3 (Cal. Ct. App. 1970).

People v. Yukl. 1975. 372 N.Y.S. 2d 313 (N. Y. Sup. Ct. 1975).

Perkins, R. M., and R. N. Boyce. 1982. Responsibility: Limitation on criminal capacity. In *Criminal Law*, 3d ed., ch. 8. Mineola, N.Y.: Foundation Press.

Powell v. Texas. 1968. 392 U.S. 514 (1968).

Raine, G. 1996. Inmates "ridiculous" lawsuits rile officials. *San Francisco Examiner* (Feb. 11): A1.

Risch, N. 1990. Genetic linkage and complex diseases, with special reference to psychiatric disorders. *Genet. Epidemiol.* 7: 3–16.

Roach v. Martin. 1985. 757 F.2d 1463 (4th Cir. 1985).

Roberts, D. E. 1991. Punishing drug addicts who have babies: Women of color, equality, and the right of privacy. *Harvard Law Rev.* 104: 1419, 1451.

Roberts, D. E. 1993. Crime, race, and reproduction. *Tulane Law Rev.* 67: 1945, 1954–1955.

Robinson v. California. 1962. 370 U.S. 660.

Sanberg, A. A., et al. 1961. An XYY human male. *Lancet* 488–489 (Aug. 21).

Sandyk, R. 1992. L-Trytophan in neuropsychiatric disorders: A review. *Int. J. Neurosci.* 67: 127–144.

Scammahorn v. State. 1987. 506 N.E.2d 1097 (Ind. 1987).

Shatzkin, K. 1996. U.S. May sue state over prison; Justice Dept. claims "Supermax" inmates' rights are violated. *Baltimore Sun* (May 8): 1A.

Skinner v. Railway Labor Executives' Association. 1989. 489 U.S. 602, 617 (1989).

Stanley v. Illinois. 1972. 405 U.S. 645, 651 (1972).

State v. Dean. 1975. 543 P.2d 425 (Ariz. 1975).

State v. Roberts. 1976. 544 P.2d 754, 758 (Wash. 1976).

State v. Ruiz. 1973. 504 P.2d 1307 (Ariz. 1973).

State v. Russell. 1991. 477 N.W.2d 886 (Minn. 1991).

Stewart, J. T. 1987. Adverse behavioral effects of amantadine therapy in Huntington's disease. *South. Med. J.* 80: 1324–1325.

Stewart, J. T., M. L. Mounts, and R. L. Clark Jr. 1987. Aggressive behavior in Huntington's disease. *J. Clin. Psychol.* 48: 106–108.

Stolberg, S. 1993. Fear clouds search for genetic roots of violence. *Los Angeles Times* (Dec. 30, 31): A1 (parts I, II).

Tarasoff v. Regents of the University of California. 1976. 551 P.2d 334 (Cal. 1976).

Taylor, L. 1982. The genetic defense. *Science Digest* 44 (Nov.).

Tenney v. State, 511 A.2d1 (Del. 1986).

Texas Criminal Procedure Code Ann. 1996. art. 37.071 §2(b)(1) (Vernon's Supp. 1996).

U.S.C.A. 1994. 18 U.S.C.A. §17 (1994).

United States v. Beck. 1979. 602 F.2d 726 (5th Cir. 1979).

United States v. Click. 1987. 807 F.2d 847 (9th Cir. 1987).

United States v. Knotts. 1983. 460 U.S. 276 (1983).

United States v. Lopez. 1971. 328 F.Supp. 1077 (E.D.N.Y. 1971).

United States v. Martinez-Fuerte. 1976. 428 U.S. 543 (1976).

United States v. Mendenhall. 1980. 446 U.S. 544 (1980).

United States v. Taylor. 1992. 956 F.2d 572, 576 n.2 (6th Cir. 1992).

Verkraik, R. 1995. It's in my genes, m'lud. *Independent* 31 (May 10).

Veronia School District 47J v. Acton, 515 U.S. 646 (1995).

Virginia Code Annotated. 1995. §19.2-310.6 (1995).

Washington, H. A. 1994. Human guinea pigs. *Emerge* (Oct.): 24–35.

Wise v. Florida. 1991. 580 So.2d 329 (Fla. 1991).

7 Behavioral Genetics and Dismantling the Welfare State

Dorothy Nelkin, Ph.D.

In her presidential address to the Behavioral Genetics Association in 1987, Sandra Scarr proclaimed that her field had arrived: there was no longer any dispute among responsible scientists or the public about the strict genetic basis of human behavior (Scarr 1987). In fact, however, there is a great deal of dispute among scientists about the importance of genes in determining complex behaviors, as we know from persistent debates over the genetic basis of violence. Yet, Scarr's claim about the public acceptance of genetic explanations appears to be true, for the idea of biological determinism has a remarkable popular appeal in American society.

In *The DNA Mystique: The Gene as a Cultural Icon,* historian Susan Lindee and I documented the popular appeal of genetic explanations in mass culture (Nelkin and Lindee 1995). We explored diverse media, including popular magazines, television sitcoms and soaps, newspaper reports, advertisements, comic books, child care books, and films, and found hundreds of articles and stories on the genetic causes of human behavior. Books on sociobiology, evolutionary psychology, and behavioral genetics—presented as the cutting edge of modern science—are instant best sellers. Included among the traits attributed to heredity in the popular media have been aggression and violence, homosexuality, exhibitionism, addiction, arson, intelligence, learning disabilities, tendency to tease, propensity for risk taking, family loyalty, religiosity, social potency, tendency to giggle, traditionalism, happiness, and zest for life.

What is the source of this appeal? Why are social problems increasingly framed in terms of the genetic predisposition of individuals to behave in certain ways? In the 1950s, explanations of human behavior—intelligence, deviance, learning ability or disability—had more to do with circumstances than susceptibilities. However, the rhetoric has changed significantly—and this, I will argue, is having significant policy implications. Framing the way we think about individual success or failure and about the sources of social problems, the ideas advanced by evolutionary psychologists and behavioral geneticists have meaning for the implementation and justification of social policy.

Historical experience has demonstrated the cultural importance of scientific ideas, especially when they coincide with prevailing social preoccupations and support existing beliefs. The scientific illumination of what is "natural" has long served to justify social policies. In the late nineteenth century, for example, the science of eugenics was premised on the notion of human improvement, an appealing factor in the cultural context of social reform in the United States. During the 1920s, eugenics complemented the social agendas of fiscal conservatives, Social Darwinists, Prohibitionists, and anti-immigration nativists, each of whom used eugenic ideas to support their political goals (Kevles 1985). Today as well genetic and evolutionary explanations appeal as a way to address the issues that trouble society: the perceived decline of the family, the problems of crime, persistent poverty, changes in the ethnic structure of the population, and the problems of the public schools.

For those concerned about changes in the family, for example, emphasizing the importance of genetic connections is an easy way to define unambiguous, solid, and immutable relationships. For those concerned about crime, explaining violence as a genetic predisposition allows blame to be placed on individuals while ignoring their social circumstances. For those concerned about the social and economic impacts of immigration, claims that there are biological distinctions between races provide an apparently scientific basis to legitimate controversial nativist social policies. And for those concerned about the problems of public schools, defining learning disabilities and behavioral disorders as biological deficiencies serves the need for efficiency and accountability.

This chapter addresses the cultural appeal of genetic explanations of behavior in the context of the political climate of the 1990s—in particular, the efforts to dismantle the welfare state. Such explanations are in effect a means to demonstrate the limits of social intervention. In a review of the fields of sociobiology and evolutionary psychology, a lawyer, Amy Wax (1996), observes that the lessons people draw from these sciences align with social conservatism in three ways: they locate the main obstacle to radical social change in the individual, not in the larger society; they suggest that traditional institutions are superior because they reflect biological endowments; and they emphasize the importance of traditional "cultural values."

I describe how claims emerging from these scientific fields are drawn into policy and legal debates to support arguments about the limits of social intervention. Much of the public discussion about the social implications of genetics has focused on the problems of employment and insurance discrimination as predictive information about future health is revealed by genetic tests

(Nelkin and Tancredi 1995; Holtzman 1989). I focus, however, on the appropriation of genetic explanations of behavior to justify a range of social policy decisions.

Biological explanations that help to identify and predict potential problems can, of course, be useful to individuals, opening the way for remedial or preventive actions. They can also provide moral relief for stigmatized conditions; that is why homosexuals welcomed research on the so-called gay gene. Theories of genetic causation are welcomed by others, such as the parents of the mentally ill, as a way to alleviate blame. However, by locating the source of social problems within the individual, theories of genetic causation also serve political agendas, for they reduce the responsibility of the state. Moreover, genetic explanations of behavior translate into moral guidelines about normal, or natural behavior. At the same time, they provide the equivalent of moral absolution, exonerating individuals by attributing antisocial acts to an independent biological force beyond the influence of volition—the DNA.

To suggest the appeal of genetic explanations of human behavior, I will draw material from two sources: the growing presence of such explanations in mass culture media, and the use of such explanations in social policy debates. In both cases, the language of genetics appeals as a way to extend the certainty and predictability of science to troubling and controversial terrains.

Explaining Antisocial Behavior

The most widely publicized research in behavioral genetics seeks to explain the causes of deviant or antisocial behavior, and especially the origins of criminal violence. Though such research is highly controversial, it has attracted enormous media attention, catering to the public fear of crime. The idea of a "criminal gene" has been the subject of numerous talk shows, cartoons, and magazine and television stories. The genetic basis of crime—the idea that criminal tendencies are inherited—has been the theme of prime time TV dramas with titles such as *Tainted Blood* or *Born to Kill*. Those who have inherited "bad genes"—so go these stories—will do violence, even when raised in ideal social environments. "Raising your child right is not enough" writes a *New York Times* journalist reporting on a teenage murderer who had been raised in a "church-going family" (Newman 1991). Another writer put it more succinctly: "Evil is embedded in the coils of chromosomes that our parents pass on to us at conception" (Franklin 1989, 36).

Also appearing in mass culture media are speculations about the policy implications of predicting genetic predisposition to violence. Genetic information, suggests the media, could be used to predict and prevent violent crime. "Rape could be reduced greatly," says a writer for the American Airlines magazine, *The American Way,* "if we had a way to determine who was biologically predisposed to it and took preemptive action" (Keehn 1992). Scientists, too, see hope in developing predictive information about criminal tendencies. Daniel Koshland, former editor of *Science,* describes a wide variety of crimes and suggests that, "When we can accurately predict future behavior, we may be able to prevent the damage" (Koshland 1992, 777).

What is the effect of pervasive messages suggesting the critical importance of genetic predisposition? Repeated media messages create the unarticulated assumptions and fundamental beliefs that underlie social policies and institutional practices as well as individual decisions. The courts, for example, are increasingly influenced by ideas of genetic causation. Biological defenses, based on the concept of genetic predisposition, are appearing in the courts because of their implications for defining the limits of criminal responsibility and free will. When geneticist Xandra Breakefield associated an extremely rare mutation in a gene for the monoamine oxidase (MAO) enzyme with the high incidence of impulsive aggression among the men in a Dutch family, she received calls from lawyers who wanted their clients tested for the defect. In Georgia, the lawyers appealing the death sentence of a murderer, Stephen Mobley, used a genetic defense to argue that Mobley was not responsible for the crime because his genes predisposed him to violence. Mobley did come from a family line that included a number of aggressive males (though some had expressed aggression in successful business ventures). The lawyers suggested this could imply a genetic predisposition to violence that precluded free will, and they asked the court to give their client a genetic test. When the court refused to pay the costs, the lawyers eventually dropped the argument, but this is one of many examples where biological defenses are becoming a means to argue for mitigating punishment (Nelkin and Tancredi 1995). Biology-based arguments, however, are malleable, and could easily be appropriated for other ends. The perception that genetic conditions are hopeless and immutable could call, for example, for permanent incarceration or even the death penalty for those with "bad" genes. Recently some states have enacted sexual predatory statutes that require "propensity hearings." Claims about genetic predisposition are of obvious interest.

Given the pressures of cost and time that currently plague the criminal justice system, genetic explanations of violent behavior conveniently fit with current ideologies about prison reform. Disillusioned with the failure of past rehabilitation schemes and pressed to save money, criminologists are leaning toward the "selective incapacitation" of prisoners instead of efforts to rehabilitate them (Jeffery, 1990). Theories of behavioral genetics can be appropriated to justify these trends. One psychologist writes, "The criminal is a different species entirely. . . . There is nothing to which to rehabilitate a criminal" (Jakes 1984, 84–85). Research funds in the field of criminology are increasingly directed toward studies of the biological cause of violent behavior.

Refuting ideas about the genetic causation of crime, biologist Herbert Needleman offers another explanation of violence that is also biology based, but links aggressive behavior to environmental sources (Needleman et al. 1996). He has studied the association between violence among youth and lead poisoning, discovering that exposure to lead can cause biological changes in the brain that result in loss of impulse control. Such mutations, Needleman argues, follow not from a genetic predisposition but from correctable environmental causes.

Just as violence is often explained in biological terms, so too is alcoholism, and this too can be appropriated to serve diverse agendas. In 1984, the Gallo wine company created the Ernest Gallo Clinic and Research Center, supporting research to identify the biological causes of alcohol abuse. In 1993, the center's scientists identified what they claimed to be a gene responsible for alcoholism. They hypothesized that this gene produced a protein that "jams the signals" warning a person to stop drinking. Those who lack this genetic warning system are prone to become alcoholics. Learning about their condition allows them to take useful precautions. However, critics of the center argue that a genetic explanation of alcoholism serves the commercial goals of the wine industry that supports the research; it locates responsibility for alcoholism, not on their product, but on the vulnerable individual's DNA (Miller 1994).

Opposing Immigration

Less widely discussed than alcoholism or criminal violence is the role of genetic arguments in current policy debates over immigration. Eugenic and evolutionary ideas were central to the debates about immigration during the early twentieth century (Kraut 1994). At that time those ideas appealed due to economic concerns—the public cost of supporting the poor, and the threat of a new and endless supply of cheap immigrant workers. Biology-based theories influenced the restrictions on immigration from central, southern, and eastern Europe that were imposed by the 1924 Immigration Act. After World War II, eugenic arguments virtually disappeared from public discourse. Today they are reappearing (in very similar terms) in the rhetoric of nativist and anti-immigration groups (Nelkin and Michaels 1996). Directed mainly toward Hispanic immigration, this rhetoric builds on assumptions about biological differences in the behavior, skills, and intelligence of different ethnic and racial groups.

The most extreme expression of genetic arguments comes from neo-Nazis, who communicate primarily through the Internet and radio talk shows. Such groups have been encouraged by ideas appearing in widely reviewed mainstream books and magazines, where the language of genetics appeals as a source of legitimacy—a way to define their agenda, not as racist, but as rational and scientific.

Nativists are using genetic assumptions in three ways: they contend that genetically determined traits are characteristic of specific racial groups; that cultures themselves are an expression of biological characteristics; and that immigration will lead to the "mongrelization" of American society, tainting racial purity and harming the gene pool. Let me provide a few examples.

The National Alliance defines itself in its talk shows and Internet communications as "the guardian of our genetic heritage—a heritage of intelligence, physical strength and beauty" (Cotten 1993). Its opposition to immigration is based on "the natural laws of heredity," and a conviction that the inferiority of some races is a "biological fact" based on evolutionary history. Coming from extremists, such views are hardly new, but they are also appearing in mainstream media from race theorists such as Charles Murray, J. Philippe Rushton, and Peter Brimelow. Brimelow, in a best selling anti-immigration book called *Alien Nation* (1995), notes that America's core comes from "European stock" (picking up on the early eugenics language of animal breeding). In *The Bell Curve* (1995, 342), Charles Murray and Richard Herrnstein argue that economic inequities are a ratification of genetic justice and insist that immigration policy must consider that Latino and black immigrants "are putting downward pressure on the distribution of intelligence. The cognitive capacity of the country is at stake." In a book published by a social science press, Rushton (1995) presents a gene-based theory of racial differences in brain and genital size based on evolutionary adaptations. Such differences, he says, call for racial selectivity in immigration.

In their efforts to deny the possibility of assimilation, these writers define culture itself as a biological phenomenon. They believe that cultures develop through evolutionary changes that express the genetic characteristics of their people. Based on a Darwinian model of world history, this view posits that some people are intrinsically backward and some nations intrinsically poor. They "possess differing degrees of evolution." Brimelow, for example, claims that the process by which nations are created are "to a considerable extent biological." He writes that the Zulu nation is prone to "natural impulsiveness and present orientation." Rushton, too, argues that people create cultures that express their genotypes; that questions of order, sociopolitical attitudes, and racial variation in skills are all rooted in genetic makeup.

The gene-based arguments of the early eugenics movement are also reappearing in concerns about "extinction," "race suicide," "dysgenesis," or a dangerous decline in the "quality" of the gene pool. "The bottom line is simple," says an Internet news group. "The USA is spiraling down the toilet of devolving dysgenesis into a third world cesspool" (Aurelius 1995). More mainstream population control advocates express similar concerns in only slightly more civil language. Garret Hardin calls immigration "passive genocide as the genes of one group replace the genes of the other" (Hardin 1995). Herrnstein and Murray worry about "dysgenic" tendencies in the reproductive patterns of today's American society.

These views enter the policy discourse through anti-immigration lobbying groups. The most influential of these, the Federation for American Immigration Reform (FAIR), is supported by the Pioneer Fund, an organization with an explicitly eugenics agenda that has also supported Rushton and Arthur Jensen's work on race and IQ. FAIR's founder, John Tanton, chair until 1987, and still on its board, publicly expressed his concerns about the "reproductive powers" of immigrants (Tanton 1988). The current director, Dan Stein, frames his opposition to immigration in economic terms and dissociates himself from the explicitly eugenic framework of the European rightists such as Le Pen. However, Stein also worries about race suicide and the future "quality of the nation" (Stein 1995).

There is nothing new in scientific research that would support these generalizations: they draw more from armchair speculations than scientific studies. However, they are gaining respectability because of a wider tendency to view human traits through what Troy Duster has called "the prism of heritability" (Duster 1990). There is a growing willingness to promulgate neo-Darwinist theories to explain why some people thrive in the competitive world of the 1990s and others do not. Scientists themselves have helped to foster the trend. In a paper written for the Marine Biological Laboratory at Woods Hole, Massachusetts, the former editor of *Science,* Daniel Koshland, argued that genetics is important in selecting people with superior skills because, "As society gets more complex, perhaps it must select for individuals more capable of coping with its complex problems" (Koshland 1988).

Explaining Social Inequities

Seeking to understand the paradox of persistent poverty in an affluent society, some social policy analysts have turned to explanations based on individual pathology. In the 1980s, a widely disseminated neoconservative critique of liberalism attacked welfare programs and blamed the problems of poverty on liberal governmental policies of social intervention (Murray 1984). Today, genetic explanations are appropriated to explain the persistence of social inequities: people are simply driven—and limited—by their genes. This is a time-worn idea. During the eugenics movement in the early part of the century, conditions such as "pauperism" were defined as "in the blood" because poverty persists in families over several generations (Kevles 1985).

In retrospect, it is easy to see the fallacies in such formulations, but similar beliefs have re-emerged in public discourse, appearing in the persistent preoccupation with what makes people different. A television newscaster described a teenager who, though raised in a poor family with no father, became the captain of his track team and won a college scholarship. "He has a quality of strength and I guess it has a genetic basis" (NBC 1988). A *Newsweek* article explained how poverty or abuse affects children differently. "Some have protective factors that serve as buffers against the risks. . . . It is the genetic luck of the draw" (Gelman 1991). The biological basis of social distinctions is the theme of *The Bell Curve* in which Herrnstein and Murray make claims for the critical importance of differential intelligence in perpetuating social class differences.

Such explanations, based on beliefs about the importance of heredity, conflict with the most basic assumptions underlying the democratic experiment in

America—the belief in the improvability, indeed the perfectibility, of human beings. They represent a remarkable change in the "bootstrap ideology" that once pervaded American folklore; neither individual actions nor social opportunity really matter if our fate lies in our genes. This is especially useful in a society that is seeking to reduce the costly social services provided by the state.

The appropriation of DNA to explain individual differences recasts common beliefs about the importance of heredity in powerful scientific terms. Science becomes a way to justify existing social categories as based on natural forces. The rich and powerful are what they are because of their genes; and so too are those who are dysfunctional. Opportunity becomes less critical than predisposition; for belief in genetic destiny implies there are natural limits constraining the individual. The moral is that no possible social system, no possible educational or nurturing plan, can change the status quo.

The policy implications of such explanations were explicit in a statement proposing new guidelines for future philanthropy from private organizations. Private philanthropy has been based on the conviction that given the opportunities provided by money, people can change. However, according to this statement—a response to *The Bell Curve*—evidence ("widely accepted by experts") about the heritability of intelligence and other behavioral characteristics is challenging this conviction. "Philanthropic efforts to help disadvantaged groups may well be thwarted to the extent that their differences are hereditary" (Lemkowitz 1994).

Explaining Educational Failures

During the 1960s, explanations for academic failure had centered on environmental sources of behavioral and learning problems—the family, the teachers, the organization of the classroom. However, in the 1980s, explanations began to draw on the biological sciences, arguing that problems were located less in a student's social situation than in the biological structure of his or her brain. These ideas have been reinforced by the *Diagnostic and Statistical Manual of Mental Disorders* (DSM), published by the American Psychiatric Association. An influential document for establishing classification and diagnostic criteria in schools and mental health institutions, the DSM has placed increasing emphasis on the definition of learning problems as developmental disturbances rather than the result of inattention or problematic classroom management.

In the educational context, convictions about the importance of genetic predisposition have policy implications especially when they conform to political and social tendencies. The generally passive attitude about the quality of education in the United States, combined with a strong desire to reduce school taxes, creates a fertile context for genetic explanations.

Focusing attention on the aberrant individual and away from the social context, genetic assumptions have strategic value as educational institutions face demands for accountability and pressures to establish rigorous classification standards. Arguments about genetically determined abilities can be used to justify the expansion of special education programs in the schools, but in the climate of cost containment, this is unlikely. More convincing are proposals such as those advanced by Herrnstein and Murray, who turn their claims about the cognitive differences in IQ into opposition to special education and affirmative action. They see an "overwhelming tilt towards enriching the education of children from the low end of the cognitive ability distribution," and they suggest that "federal funds now so exclusively focused on the disadvantaged should be reallocated to programs for the gifted" (Herrnstein and Murray 1994, 419).

In a practical expression of these ideas, members of a taxpayer's association in a Long Island, New York, community used genetic arguments in their effort to reduce local school taxes. In 1994, they campaigned against their school district's program of special education classes for learning-disabled children by arguing that such disabilities are of genetic origin. That being the case, they concluded, responsibility should fall to the medical system, not to the schools.

Enhancing Family Values

Finally, genetic assumptions are entering social policy debates about the family, supporting the rhetoric about "family values." The family increasingly appears in popular culture and political rhetoric as a troubled institution, threatened by feminism, divorce, working mothers, alternative partnerships, gay rights, and the complex arrangements enabled by new reproductive technologies. Though many of these trends are hardly new, the family today seems to be in a special state of crisis, and genetic ideas are appropriated as a comfortable, that is, "natural" way to deal with domestic problems. The importance of genetic connections—of what may be called the "molecular family"—has become a pervasive theme in soap operas, women's magazines, and other vehicles of popular culture, and it is also appearing to guide decisions in family courts.

The molecular family, centering on the dyad of biological parent and child, is based on the cultural expectation that a biological entity can determine emotional connections and social bonds—that genetic connections somehow offer a uniquely reliable basis for the perpetuation of family values. DNA seems to ground family relationships in a stable and well-defined unit, providing the individual with indisputable roots that are more reliable than the ephemeral ties of love, marital vows, or shared experiences. Genes, after all, create ties that can never be severed, and they validate the individual as genetically placed in an unambiguous relationship to others.

In popular theories of evolutionary psychology and sociobiology, the idea that genetic bonds are truly lasting is even used to naturalize infidelity through claims about the importance of maximizing future genetic relationships. In 1994, *Time* published a cover story about Robert Wright's book *The Moral Animal* (1994). The cover proclaimed "Infidelity: It May Be in Our Genes." Wright had provided an evolutionary account of the development of social conventions such as marriage. These conventions, he wrote, were based on norms that evolved over time to efficiently propagate genes. However, they can be destroyed by policies based on moral neutrality and tolerance. Thus, he suggests, state welfare programs are bound to weaken the institution of marriage among the poor.

Genetic assumptions dominate stories about infertility, adoption, and the search for biological roots, and they have had considerable policy influence. Today, in most states, adoption records, which were once concealed, have been opened in order to facilitate the adoptee's search for biological "roots." Custody or surrogacy decisions are often framed in family courts as conflicts between genetic and social connections. In custody cases, judges are interpreting genetic connections as central to personal identity, and invoking theories of behavioral genetics to explain their decisions. For example, in a California case over the custody of a child born in a surrogacy arrangement, the judge called the surrogate mother a "genetic hereditary stranger" and cited studies of identical twins to justify the need for placing the child with the biological mother (*Johnson v. Calvert* 1990).

Other courts have drawn on science to argue the importance of "genetic rights." While the outcome of such cases varies, the importance of genetic connections is becoming integrated into judicial assumptions about parenthood—sometimes overriding the traditional guidelines based on the best interests of the child (Dolgin 1993).

Responsibility and Blame

This analysis of popular and policy discourse suggests how scientific concepts concerning the heritability of behavior have been translated into a rhetoric of responsibility and blame. This use of genetic explanations to shift responsibility is taking place in other policy arenas as well. Cancer is increasingly defined as a genetic disease—as an inherited predisposition. Though cancer is indeed a genetic disease in the sense that it involves gene mutations, not all types of cancer are inherited. Environmental influences are responsible for most mutations. However, the redefinition of cancer as a genetic disease shifts responsibility away from industry and regulators. Thus, just as Gallo Wine is supporting research on alcoholism, so the tobacco industry is supporting research on the molecular basis of the causes of lung cancer, hoping, according to critics, to sow doubt about the dangers of smoking (Cohen 1996).

Similarly, the defendants in toxic tort cases are looking at the genetic predisposition of plaintiffs as a way to shift blame. In a products liability suit, for example, a plaintiff blamed his birth defects on *in utero* exposure to toxics at the plant where his mother worked. The defendant, however, claimed that a genetic disorder had caused the defects, not exposure to toxics (*Severson v. KTI Chemicals*, 1994). In a similar liability case, a company tried to compel a plaintiff to take a test for fragile X syndrome, insisting that his disability was not caused by toxic substances, but was innate (Paul Billings, personal communication, July 17, 1996).

On the other hand, genetic explanations of mental illness have changed the rhetoric of responsibility and blame in this area in ways that are often useful. The National Alliance for the Mentally Ill (NAMI), for example, welcomed, indeed supported, research on the genetics of mental illness because it relieved parents of the mentally ill from blame. However, there is growing concern among NAMI members as well as among other disability groups that genetic explanations could also devalue the disabled by defining them as intrinsically flawed. Families could be blamed in different ways—that is, for passing on "bad" genes—and they fear that belief in genetic causation will limit their reproductive freedom.

Biology-based explanations of mental illness have dramatically changed the treatment of the mentally ill. The attribution of pathological behavior to biological causes has turned psychiatrists into psychopharmacologists, for drugs are now the central tool of therapy. In many cases this has been useful. The changes have been partly driven by progress in the scientific understanding of mental illness and the proven therapeutic effectiveness of certain drugs. However, the changes are also a response to economic pressures for rapid and cost-effective treatment brought about by changes in reimbursement strategies and the need to enhance efficiency and control costs. How do genetic explanations and the economic pressures faced by health-care institutions intersect? How often are biological explanations used to justify cost-effective therapies when analytic methods are more appropriate?

As cost containment becomes the primary goal of the health-care delivery system, people with chronic and costly diseases are finding themselves excluded from benefits as they quickly exceed the caps permitted for their condition. This is particularly devastating for those with genetic conditions. In the military, for example, servicemen who discover they have a genetic disease while in the service have been discharged without benefits on the reasoning that it was a preexisting condition (Billings, personal communication). As more conditions—especially those in the complex area of human behavior—are defined as genetic, more people will be excluded from social services.

Regardless of Scarr's enthusiastic claims in 1987, behavioral genetics remains controversial. Many critics have questioned the motivation behind efforts to measure the relative effects of nature and nurture on human behavior. Psychologist Douglas Wahlsten writes that "the only practical application of a heritability coefficient is to predict the results of a program of selective breeding" (Wahlsten 1990, 119). Discussions of the genetics of crime have invariably provoked disputes such as the much-publicized controversy over a 1995 conference organized by the University of Maryland to explore theories about the genetic basis of criminal behavior.

When faced with such criticism, advocates of behavioral genetics—and they often assume the role of advocates as well as researchers—deny they are genetic determinists. Of course, they say, the social environment matters. However, the terms they use suggest their deterministic assumptions; they refer to behavioral traits as "hard wired," the body as a "program," and people as "read-outs" of their genes. We are, writes Robert Wright, "pushed and pulled by feelings designed to propagate our genes" (Wright, 1994). Geneticists place great stake in the power of genetic prediction: the genome is a "Delphic oracle"; "Our fate lies in our genes."

When confronted with the abuse of their science, as in cases of genetic discrimination or the situations I have described, scientists often blame the media or the uninformed public. Claiming the moral neutrality of science, they insist that their job is to do good research; the use of their work is not their responsibility (comments of David Goldman, M.D., July 17, 1996). However, scientists, concerned about obtaining public funds, encourage the appropriation of their work through their repeated claims about its social importance. At the very least, they have the responsibility to minimize the possibilities of misinterpretation of work that is highly subject to abuse.

Drawing from several different policy areas, I have suggested the appeal of genetic explanations as a scientific justification of various social, political, and economic agendas. Such explanations are easily appropriated—and often in contradictory ways. They can be used to justify racial biases, to reinforce social divisions, and to support ideas about "family values." They can be used to deflect the blame for social problems onto the individual or to exonerate an individual as blameless in the face of biological predispositions. Genetic explanations can be used to absolve the state from responsibility for providing social services, but also to absolve the individual from responsibility for his actions— "It's all in the genes." Recourse to genetics can express a sense of fatalism—"the luck of the draw" or a moral judgment—there are good and bad genes. Claims about genetic inferiority or the "natural" distinctions between racial groups can be used to clothe racist theories in the neutral garb of scientific discourse, and to label certain people as likely burdens on the state.

Behavioral genetics is in vogue these days—just as eugenics was in the 1920s—in part because it suits the political context, providing justification for social policies and legitimation for political goals. It is interesting that at a time when government funding of most areas of research is drastically declining, the field of genetics is enjoying continuing and even expanding congressional support. It is revealing to follow the uncritical and unquestioned adoption of genetic language and assumptions in a wide range of popular media. As these assumptions become broadly accepted in American culture, they are influencing the decisions of schools, courts, health-care professions, and other institutions because they seem to serve short-term economic and administrative needs. Indeed, the policy significance of genetic explanations of human behavior is likely to grow as an expanding science meets the shifting social agendas of the 1990s.

References

Aurelius, M. 1995. Internet newsgroup posting in alt. politics. nationalism. white, June 17.

Brimelow, P. 1995. *Alien Nation.* New York: Random House.

Cohen, J. 1996. Tobacco money lights up a debate, *Science* 272 (26 Apr.): 488–494.

Cotten, R. 1993. American dissident voices, September 11 (Minuteman Books).

Dolgin, J. 1993. Just a gene: Judicial assumptions about parenthood. *UCLA Law Rev.* 40: 637–694.

Duster, T. 1990. *Backdoor to Eugenics.* New York: Routledge.

Franklin, D. 1989. What a child is given. *New York Times Magazine* (3 Sept.): 36.

Gelman, D. 1991. The miracle of resiliency. *Newsweek Special Issue* (summer): 44–47.

Hardin, G. 1995. Commentary. *Chronicles: A Magazine of American Culture* (July): 178.

Herrnstein, R., and C. Murray. 1994. *The Bell Curve.* New York: Free Press.

Holtzman, N. 1989. *Proceed with Caution: Predicting Genetic Risks in the Recombinant DNA Era.* Baltimore: Johns Hopkins University Press.

Jake's Page. 1984. Exposing the criminal mind. *Science* 84 (Sept.): 84–85.

Jeffery, C. R. 1990. *Criminology.* Englewood Cliffs, N.J.: Prentice-Hall.

Johnson V. Calvert, 1990. Nos. x-633190 and AD-57638 (Cal. App. Dep't. Super. Oct. 22, 1990).

Keehn, J. 1992. The long arm of the gene. *American Way* (15 Mar.): 36–38.

Kevles, D. 1985. *In the Name of Eugenics.* New York: Knopf.

Koshland, D. 1988. The future of biological research. *MBL-Science* 3: 10–13.

Koshland, D. 1992. Elephants, monstrosities and the law. *Science* 255 (14 Feb.): 777.

Kraut, A. 1994. *Silent Travelers.* New York: Basic Books.

Lemkowitz, L. 1994. "What philanthropy can learn from *The Bell Curve.*" Hudson Institute (Nov. 29).

Miller, M. 1994. In vino veritas. *Wall Street Journal* (June 8).

Murray, C. 1984. *Losing Ground.* New York: Basic Books.

NBC. 1988. *Kids and Stress.* News special (Apr. 25).

Needleman, H. L., J. A. Riess, M. Y. Tobin, G. E. Biesecker, and J. B. Greenhouse. 1996. Bone lead levels and delinquent behavior. *J. Am. Med. Assoc.* 275: 363–369.

Nelkin, D., and M. S. Lindee. 1995. *The DNA Mystique: The Gene as a Cultural Icon.* New York: Freeman.

Nelkin, D., and M. Michaels. 1998. Biological categories and social controls. *Soc. Policy* 18: 33–62.

Nelkin, D., and L. Tancredi. 1995. *Dangerous Diagnostics: The Social Power of Biological Information.* Chicago: University of Chicago Press.

Newman, M. 1991. Raising children right isn't always enough. *New York Times* (22 Dec.).

Rushton, J. P. 1994. *Race, Evolution, and Behavior.* New Brunswick, N.J.: Transaction Books.

Scarr, S. 1987. Three cheers for behavioral genetics. *Behav. Genet.* 17(3): 219–228.

Severson v. KTI Chemicals. 1994. Nonrecorded case S040488, Supreme Court of California. Appeal denied June 22, 1994.

Stein, D. 1995. Letter. *Policy Review* (Jan.).

Tanton, J. 1988. *Arizona Republic,* quoted in James Crawford, *Hold Your Tongue.* Reading, Mass.: Addison Wesley, 1992, 151.

Wahlsten, D. 1990. Insensitivity of the analysis of variance to heredity-environment interaction. *Behav. Brain Sci.* 13: 109–161.

Wax, A. L. 1996. Against nature. *University of Chicago Law Rev.* 63: 307–359.

Wright, R. 1994. *The Moral Animal.* New York: Pantheon.

8 The Social Consequences of Genetic Disclosure

Troy Duster, Ph.D.

The social consequences of disclosure of genetic information are as varied as the societies in which such disclosure occurs and depend on the local social meanings attached to the information disclosed. For example, at one extreme, the simple knowledge of whether a fetus has the Y chromosome (which determines sex) can be, and has been fatal for the fetus. Long before the advent of prenatal detection technologies, preference for a male child in India was so great that a notable fraction of the population practiced infanticide of newborn females. Once technologies for determining sex became available, the quest for "disclosure" took an ominous turn. An excerpt from a general letter sent out in early 1982 by Bhandari Hospital in India, states: "Most prospective clients in quest of a male child, as the social set-up of India demands, keep on giving birth to a number of female children, which in a way not only enhances the increasing population, but leads to a chain reaction of many social, economic, and mental stresses on these families. . . . Antenatal sex determination has come to our rescue and can help in keeping some check over the population as well as give relief to the couples requiring male children" (*India Today* 1982).

In 1971, India enacted the Medical Termination of Pregnancy Act, which stipulates that a woman can be given an abortion only if there is a life-threatening situation or grave injury to her physical or mental health. Amniocentesis began in India in 1974, at the Human Cytogenetics Unit in New Delhi. Early reports indicated that the test was being used less often to detect birth defects than to determine the sex of the fetus. The Indian medical establishment, the Indian Council of Medical Research, requested that this practice be discontinued. While the New Delhi clinic complied with the request for the most part, private clinics sprang up in several cities to respond to requests for prenatal knowledge of a fetus's sex. Within two years, more than a dozen such places were in operation in India.

So many Indian physicians ignored the 1971 law prohibiting abortion for sex selection that the government began a new round of hearings in the late

1980s to consider legislation restricting the use of new technologies to determine the sex of the fetus.[1] In 1988, the state of Maharastra introduced legislation to ban the use of prenatal diagnosis for sex determination after a report estimated that approximately 78,000 fetuses were aborted in India between 1978 and 1982 (Rao 1988). Rao reports on a study in Bombay in which, of 8,000 abortions, 7,997 were female fetuses (Rao 1986).

In August 1994, the Indian Parliament passed a new law that stiffened the penalties for screening the fetus to determine sex. It provides for three years imprisonment and a fine of approximately $320 for administering a test with the sole purpose of prenatal sex determination. The law, however, applies only to clinics. The use of mobile ultrasound units renders the law practically meaningless, and the practice of prenatal sex discrimination continues at such a high rate that in Haryana, a populous northern state, the sex ratio is an astonishingly low 874 females to every 1,000 males.[2]

"Individual Decision" or Unexamined Group Pattern?

It is clear from these examples of sex preferences in India that what appear to be individual familial choices are actually often better understood as socially patterned practices that reflect social and cultural authority. In early 1994, *Nature* published an article titled "China's Misconception of Eugenics," pointing out that the Chinese government's policy of trying to prohibit couples with certain diseases from procreating had a distasteful eugenic quality (*Nature*, 1994, 1). Although the article contained a forthright denunciation of the use of state power to prohibit individuals from procreating, it implied that an individual decision to interrupt a pregnancy is necessarily "voluntary." "China's plans for eugenics must be judged by the degree to which they interfere with people's wishes; they may not differ much from programmes followed elsewhere but compulsion will make them unacceptable" (1994, 1).[3]

There is considerable evidence to support the observation that what we in Western societies characterize as individual decisions are on closer inspection (as with sex selection in India) very remarkably socially patterned. The situation is not reducible to an either/or formulation. A continuum is a better analytic device for arraying strategies and options, from individual choice to embedded but powerful social pressures (stigma and ridicule), to economic pressures (loss of health insurance or the inability to obtain such insurance), to the coercive power of the state to penalize.

While it is true that individuals make those choices, they do so in an unsubtly coercive social and economic context. To characterize such choices as voluntary is to so stretch the meaning of the term as to make it useless. While this is relatively obvious when we look at other societies, it is substantially obscured in our own because "individual choice" is deeply embedded in cultural assumptions that we take for granted.

Prenatal determination is but one of the developments of the past quarter century that has affected reproductive decision making. The disclosure that a fetus has a life-threatening disorder such as beta-thalassemia or cystic fibrosis can result in social ostracism both for the affected person and for parents and siblings. Moreover, depending on whether health care is available, the social consequences can be economically crippling. For this reason, disclosure of the existence of a genetic disorder can produce dissimulation and even outright lying to prospective mates or health-care providers; it certainly affects relations with those who are in a position to authorize payments for health care. In addition, for many genetic disorders, the affected person may choose to avoid disclosure to an employer or a prospective employer for fear that the information will negatively affect employment opportunities.

Although the focus of this chapter is on genetic information purveyed by health professionals who collect, interpret, and distribute such information, much genetic information is disclosed all the time, with important social consequences. One does not need to conduct a test at the molecular level for such disclosure to occur. Knowledge about a family's health history will suffice.

Contemporary America: General Acceptance and Specific Fears of Disclosure

At the moment, the fear of disclosure of genetic information is not very high in the general population of the United States, at least as measured by the most extensive national survey on the topic, conducted by the Lou Harris poll for the March of Dimes in the spring of 1992. From that survey, Harris concluded that nearly 60 percent of the American population believed that "if someone is a carrier of a defective gene or has a genetic disease, then someone deserves to know about it." Of those who believe that someone else deserves to know, 98 percent said a spouse or a prospective marriage partner deserves to know, and most remarkably, 58 percent thought that an insurer should know; 33 percent said that an employer should know. The poll also included an important caveat. While Americans are generally positive about the new genetic technologies and their potential uses, 70 percent of Americans admit to "knowing very little" about either genetic testing or gene therapy. (Drawn from a summary of the poll's findings.)

In families where there has actually been a diagnosis of a genetic disorder, there is a tendency to be far more skeptical, far more suspicious of insurance companies and secretive about disclosing this information even to other members of the extended family; certainly there is less likelihood of providing such information to employers. The March of Dimes survey tapped into the general population's relatively benign view of disclosure, a direct function of the public's lack of contact with the real problems of disclosure of genetic information. In contrast, those "in the experience" tend to express the opposite views about such disclosure, and see it as anything but benign. In other words, people who have had the experience of being in a family in which a genetic disorder has been diagnosed have views diametrically opposed to those responding to an abstract hypothetical question anonymously posed in a fifteen-minute telephone interview for a national opinion survey (Duster and Beeson 1997).

The two most common inherited, potentially lethal, single-gene disorders in the United States are sickle cell anemia (SC) and cystic fibrosis (CF). While cystic fibrosis occurs primarily among Americans of (North) European descent, sickle cell disease occurs primarily among Americans of (West) African descent. Genetic testing is available for both disorders. In the summer of 1992, I was part of a team of social scientists that embarked on a study to determine communication patterns about the two genetic disorders in families where one of these diseases had been detected. We noted that this would provide a unique opportunity to compare the variable penetration and meaning of genetic information in two populations differentiated by the socially designated categories of "race."

The research began in the summer of 1992 and originated in clinical settings, but fanned out to support groups and advocacy organizations serving individuals and families with a special interest or concern about either sickle cell anemia or cystic fibrosis. The research team has completed the study, with 369 interviews of men and women who have, or who have had, a person with one of these conditions (or in some cases a known carrier) in their family.

Since the purpose of the project was to reveal cultural and social-structural variations in perspectives, the interviewing strategies were designed to minimize semantic structuring of responses. We also attempted to avoid the impression that we were testing knowledge, because that sets up an entirely different dynamic in which respondents tend to reveal less personal information. Interviewing was designed to elicit narratives relevant to six general topic areas. Within these six areas we developed a series of open-ended probes to explore the specific terrain relevant to each interviewee:

1. History of personal experience with CF/SC. The interviewer began by asking how respondents first learned about CF or SC and then explored their entire personal history, probing for appropriate details, including thoughts, feelings, and behavior in response to specific events.

2. Perspectives on the disease. We explored the respondents' beliefs about the meaning of the disorder in the lives of those affected and what they think is the best response to the threat of the disease, including their perspectives on prevention and treatment.

3. Genetic testing. We determined whether respondents were aware that testing is available and how they felt about carrier testing and prenatal diagnosis.

4. Family communication. We asked about family members' responses to CF or SC and carrier testing—whether they discussed it, and, if so, how it came up, and what was said. We also asked about grandparents and about differences in responses between men and women.

5. Communication with friends and acquaintances. We asked respondents if they talked with people outside the family about CF or SC, and under what conditions and how they perceived the responses of others.

6. Health care. We asked what was their main health-care concern for themselves and their family. We asked what, if anything, they would change about their health care and whether they had any concerns related to health insurance or coverage.

The interviews averaged about an hour and a half in length. During the initial focus on the personal experience of the respondents, the interviewers had the task of gaining the trust of the respondent and shifting the context from a formal, technical, and impersonal exchange to a more intimate one. We found that when confronted with the issue of genetic disease, particularly by university researchers, our respondents often began by engaging in a somewhat formal and impersonal discourse. Our probes encouraged them to go beyond this "official presentation of self" and to reveal the experience of their private worlds. These personal accounts are often more emotionally charged and inconsistent with the frontstage, public exchanges. It is from this interplay of front- and backstage discourses by family members that the current analysis emerges.

Some Relevant Findings

Our study determined that survey findings on "general attitudes toward genetic testing" of the general public are completely invalid when we turn to families where a genetic disorder, or even where being a carrier of a gene for a genetic disorder, has been detected. In the general population there is a tendency for an uncritical acceptance of the idea that the technology is beneficial, and that there is little to fear from employers or health insurance companies. In our study, however, overwhelming concern about both job insecurity and the potential for insurance cancellation made more than two-thirds of our subjects wary about disclosing the existence of the genetic character of their disease to any but close friends. Often they failed to disclose this fact even to extended family members. Even more striking, it is not unusual for siblings and others in the immediate family not to be informed of the genetic circumstances (disease or carrier status) (Duster and Beeson, 1997).

Disclosure has remarkably different consequences for different members of the family. We found a pattern in which teenagers are the most likely members of the family to want to conceal, or at least not publicly disclose their condition. Mothers (as caregivers), on the other hand, were most likely to want to disclose the condition of their child to schoolteachers and other potential caregivers. This sets up a dynamic of internal conflict in which different members of the family take sides on the level and degree of appropriate disclosure.

It should now be clear that any attempt to map out or assess the social consequences of the disclosure of genetic information takes us down complicated and winding roads. One way to make sense of all the complexities and contingencies is to develop a taxonomic system. This taxonomy moves from (1) the affected individual, to (2) the family and/or primary caretakers of the affected individual, to (3) the existing social category in which the affected individual already fits, to (4) the creation of new social categories and experiences into which the individual did not realize (before genetic testing and disclosure) that he or she would be suddenly catapulted. This set of categories is not intended to be exhaustive, but rather to suggest a strategy for developing an overview of the different kinds and levels of social concerns that attend the disclosure of genetic information obtained from the new molecular technologies.

Genetic Disease as "Socially Owned"
by the Affected Social Group

Genetic diseases often have a peculiar feature that results in a distinctive social consequence. Unlike cancer, tuberculosis, or the flu; and unlike smallpox, diabetes, or heart disease, genetic diseases for which testing and screening are likely to be available tend to cluster in populations that have already existing social categories based on ethnicity, race, gender, and sometimes language and culture. Societies are stratified internally and externally. Whatever other disagreements social scientists may have about the nature and character of social and economic organizations, no one contests this feature of all social orders, or of the "world order," new or old. Moreover, inside every society there are systems of stratification by age and sex, spiritual or intellectual power, and lineage and property.

These fundamental truths apply to the study of genetic diseases and to the study of the social consequences of the disclosure of those diseases. This is because some groups come to sense and feel their "ownership" of a disease precisely because it afflicts them more than any other group. For example, Tay-Sachs is a disease that primarily afflicts the Ashkenazi Jewish population. In the United States, sickle cell anemia is a genetic disease associated primarily with African Americans. The social, political, and economic status of a group affects the way in which its members sense or feel symbolically connected with a disease. A case at an Oakland hospital in the 1970s illustrates this. A mother reported that her son had "leukemia," not sickle cell anemia. Her genetic counselor knew that she understood the difference. When pressed on the matter of why she told people that the diagnosis was leukemia, she indirectly acknowledged that it was because she felt better if her son had a "higher status disease." (Based on research by the author.)

The ethnic distribution of genetic disorders is important. It is the foundation on which the social organization of real genetic screening programs are developed, and also provides the guideposts for gene therapy research. A recent example is the "ownership" of beta-thalassemia, originally termed "Cooley's anemia" and associated mainly with peoples from the Mediterranean region, primarily from southern Italy. However, in the past decade, with scores of thousands of immigrants from Southeast Asia, China, and Singapore entering the United States, we have discovered that the thalassemias, both beta and alpha, are showing up in Chinese, Vietnamese, and other ethnic groups from these regions, in far greater proportion than was previously known.[4]

It is possible to see political mobilization of blacks and Jews and Italians around a disorder that is "their own." A very different dimension of the social landscape of identity emerges when a genetic screen is developed that does not coincide with already established social groupings. As noted, when there is overlap with social categories, there is the likely formation of interest groups and increased social awareness and capacity for political mobilization. Yet, the social effects are also significant when there is no overlap between the genetic screen and socially identifiable groupings. There is some evidence that people of northern European ancestry, among them northern Germans, Danes, Swedes, and Norwegians, are at much greater risk for an inborn deficiency of serum alpha$_1$-antitrypsin, and are vulnerable to dust and chemical agents in the industrial workplace, which could trigger emphysema and chronic bronchitis (Lappé 1988).

If a genetic screening program were developed for this condition, a social analyst would have a solid basis for predicting a quite different pattern of mobilization than we have seen for sickle cell, Tay-Sachs, or beta-thalassemia. European Americans of north German and variable Scandinavian ancestry do not comprise a social group identifiable and known to each other. At the workplace they are far too isolated and fragmented for interest groups to form. When a small percentage of them is identified as vulnerable to emphysema because of a genetically related deficiency, neither the workers as a collectivity nor the individuals identified will see it as being in their interest to mobilize as a group. The victims will be seen as isolated and particular cases with a personal problem (Draper 1991).

Rather than seeing a social reaction to the new genetic screen (as with African Americans over sickle cell), the wave of the next period could well be the passive, individual acceptance of a "personal" problem of a genetic deficiency that does not permit one to work in certain jobs.

The Affected Individual

There are two important positive effects of disclosure on the affected individual. First, for the newborn, the disclosure can be life-saving, and certainly life-exceeding. In the case of sickle cell anemia, for example, if the family and attending medical caregivers do not know that the newborn has the disease, months and even years can pass during which symptomatic conditions are not appropriately treated. A physician may misdiagnose the painful crises occasioned by the sickling of the blood in joints and organs.

A second kind of positive effect occurs when an affected individual is given information about his or her genetic makeup, permitting an alteration in lifestyle and life choices that can extend and enhance the quality of life. Chronic obstructive pulmonary diseases such as emphysema, asthma, and bronchitis are the eleventh leading cause of years of potential life lost in the United States. It is fairly well established that genetic factors play an important role in determining age at onset of these diseases and their severity. Individuals who are homozygous for alpha$_1$-antitrypsin deficiency are at greater risk for these lung diseases. That risk is greatly exacerbated by smoking, or by being in an environment with high levels of dust, welding fumes, and a number of other substances. Smoking is regarded as a dominant factor, and contributes as much as 50 percent to the known excess risk, although the interaction of smoking with other factors is not well understood.

Lappé (1988) argued that genetic screening for susceptibility to chronic lung disease is a worthwhile project. He bases his judgment on a careful reading of material on the interaction between susceptibility and environmental hazards, such as excessive dust in the environment, and smoking. Lappé's argument is that people who are at higher risk should be informed so that they can adjust their personal behaviors and lifestyles to reduce the possibility of disease. With the focus on the individual, Lappé is compelling. So long as it remains a matter of personal choice and lifestyle, this kind of genetic screening is uncontroversial. However, when it comes to earning a livelihood, the argument about the consequences of disclosure at the worksite is heavily saturated with political and economic ideology. However well-intentioned the motives, an orientation toward genetic susceptibility can easily begin to dominate our ways of thinking about disease prevention, until it becomes the only way we think about the problem.

An individual may also experience powerful negative consequences from the disclosure of certain kinds of genetic information, depending on the social context of that disclosure. Most genetic diseases have "variable expressivity." Two people with a diagnosis at the molecular level of sickle cell anemia may have very different health outcomes. The first person might live to be sixty years of age, with a relatively full capacity to pursue a normal life, albeit with monitoring, treatment, and some adjustments to lifestyle. The second person might live to be only thirty, with severe pain during much of his or her life that is debilitating and makes it difficult to work steadily.

Given this situation, if and when a genetic professional is about to disclose the existence of a disease to an individual, there are two difficult choices of what to communicate. First, if the disclosure takes into account the wide band of possibilities for symptoms and survival, the individual is placed into a deep existential quandary as to what course of action to take. If, on the other hand, the genetic professional only informs the affected individual about a narrow band of possibilities for the future, that person may act in a fatalistic manner that is unwarranted by the uncertainty in the possibilities of expression of the disease.

An affected individual faces a different set of consequences when late-onset diseases are disclosed socially. The uncertainty that the affected individual faces may extend to family and friends. Indeed, the disclosure of a genetic basis for a disease to his or her social circles limits the freedom of an individual to make decisions that might increase his or her levels of sociability (marriage, children, extended family); these, in turn, are known to affect longevity. I am describing here a spiral effect of social disclosure that can, and often does, affect the health status of the individual, usually negatively.

Genetic Disclosure and the Family Unit

Public support for genetic research rests on the conviction that the resulting knowledge will provide significant benefits to individuals and to the general public health, a position expressed frequently in the media, as well as in the scientific and health policy literature. It has fueled the proliferation of various forms of genetic testing, and led to increasing numbers of North Americans being encouraged to integrate genetic information into their marriage decisions and reproductive lives (Holtzman 1997; Nelkin and Lindee 1995). This focus on selection of a mate and reproduction is a result of the fact that "no effective interventions are yet available to improve the outcome of most inherited diseases" (Holtzman and Watson, 1997, xi).

Very little research has examined what it means for individuals and families to integrate genetic information into their personal relationships. Most of the studies on genetic testing or the social implications of genetic advances consist of either opinion polls of the general population or interviews with patients in medical settings about their preferences. We still know relatively little about how people respond to genetic issues in the context of family and intimate relationships. Our study attempted to address how families in which genetic risk is known to exist respond to information about this risk.[5]

Family Unity

The family is by definition a collective. When information about deleterious genes is introduced, the character of that collectivity is altered, if not threatened. This is because deleterious genes never exist without bodies. Not only are they embodied, but they are unequally distributed among individuals who in some cases previously saw their membership in the family as something they shared equally with other family members. In those circumstances, a previously shared legacy is suddenly redefined in a way that emphasizes differences among family members, identifying some as having fundamental "defects," and as potentially "dangerous" to their own offspring. Meanwhile other members are certified as free of such liabilities—or at least are ignorant of those liabilities. This introduces classifications into the family that, however practical, are likely to be disruptive of previous relationships. The sensitivity family members have to these relational concerns is often interpreted from a biomedical or psychological perspective as "denial" of biomedical risk, particularly if it results in the failure to integrate genetic information into selection of a partner or reproductive planning. Yet such an orientation "denies" another fundamental social reality, the overwhelming importance of the family bond.

While genetic disease has long been known to exist, most health problems have been understood to be the result of threats from outside the family. Genetic disease, on the other hand, identifies a child's parent(s) as the source of the problem. Indeed, children sometimes refer to their condition as "a disease my parents gave me." When the source of a disease is found in parents' biological makeup, issues of guilt and blame surface. These feelings are typically displayed inadvertently rather than deliberately. A mother of a child with sickle cell disease was more explicit in voicing these feelings than some others when she stated: "I feel responsible and his dad feels the same way. It's like we have done something. We have shamed ourselves real bad, but you just have to deal with it. Society puts people down about a whole lot of things. I feel they look upon me as though I'm nasty. You know, they don't take kindly when you do something to a child. It's just bad."

Fathers have special difficulty accepting their role in their child's disorder. This even leads some to question whether they are in fact the biological father. Men more frequently reject the basic tenets of Mendelian genetics: i.e, they are far more likely than women to assert that "it couldn't have come from my side." A more constructive response was expressed by one father who refused to have his identity spoiled by genetic information. He noted, "What makes me a good parent is not whether or not my child is perfect, but what I'm able to do to help her."

The opportunities for casting blame are more apparent in the case of grandparents, who are less obviously implicated in their grandchild's condition. The neutral, technical purpose of testing them is to determine which branch of the family is at greatest risk. Nonetheless, testing invariably turns out to be a source of considerable distress for grandparents. Their first reaction to the news of a genetic disease is usually to deny that any such condition has ever existed on their side of the family. In one case the grandparent who was tested and found not to be a carrier was sworn to secrecy by her spouse, thereby nullifying the purpose of her test. Many resist testing because they anticipate difficulty living with the knowledge that they contributed, however innocently, to their grandchild's illness. As one grandmother asked: "Whose fault was it? Was it mine or my husband's? . . . I'd like to know which one—who carries the gene; my husband or I. But on the other hand, maybe it's good I don't know."

Our data suggest that these feelings of blame and shame for being what several families call "the culprit," will proliferate as we increase our capacity to identify a particular "imperfection" via genetic analysis. A sense of responsibility for a child's suffering is something few parents or grandparents can treat with neutrality, particularly when so much energy is focused on identifying the source of a disease. Humans *insist* on giving meaning to dramatic personal news. Probability theory does not provide that meaning.

While there is a full range of responses, a diagnosis of sickle cell or cystic fibrosis is typically received as devastating news. Family members repeatedly reported being told that their child will not live to adulthood and being given other similar prognoses that have very often proven unduly pessimistic. In one family we interviewed an adult who as a child (with asthma and allergies) was misdiagnosed with CF. This diagnosis caused her mother to give up hope for her daughter's future. Today, the adult daughter is very resentful that major decisions were made about her life under the erroneous assumption that she would die young: "It very much affected my relationship with her [her mother]. She was always acting like I was going to die and she made decisions about my life as if I was about to die all the time."

This case is of interest because even though the diagnosis eventually was proven incorrect, its social consequences remained significant. We have found adults with mild cases of CF or SC who were grateful they were not diagnosed sooner, because they managed to receive symptomatic treatment while living a "more normal life" and maintaining an "unspoiled" social identity.

As noted above, the knowledge that one is a carrier of a potentially fatal genetic disorder takes on particular significance when it occurs in young adulthood during or prior to the quest for a life partner. Medically this is one of the least controversial uses of genetic testing. Respondents may claim to be in favor of the idea that carriers should have their partners tested. However, when they describe their actual behavior and the behavior of other family members, it becomes clear that there is a strong undercurrent of resistance to carrier testing. While only a minority of respondents are actively outspoken in their objections, there are more frequent, implicit indications of discomfort with this concept—such as the failure to take any action, even a telephone call, to inquire about how testing might be done.

When carrier testing is done, it is usually as a result of encouragement from a health provider. Only rarely is testing done at the instigation of family members themselves. We were able to locate only two individuals out of forty-four known carriers in our sample who were identified as a result of genetic testing rather than as a result of giving birth to an affected child. Five other individuals tested proved not to be carriers. Two of those tested are a young couple, both of whom have CF in their families. They resisted suggestions by their mothers to be tested prior to marriage, because they did not want their genetic status to influence their choice of a partner, but agreed under family pressure to be tested after marriage. Since neither turned out to be a carrier, it is unclear what their response to positive results in both of them would have been. Respondents in both sickle cell and cystic fibrosis samples find carrier testing an uncomfortable fit with the ideology of romantic love.

There is considerable evidence that even when individuals have been tested and are found to be carriers (often this occurs at birth in the case of sickle cell disease), it does not necessarily lead an individual to integrate this knowledge into the selection of a partner or decisions about childbearing. These findings support a recent analysis by Hill (1994, 29–47), who also found widespread resistance to integrating sickle cell testing into selection of a mate. She describes this response in the African American communities she studied as "obfuscation of SCD medical knowledge" and attributes it to SC's threat to motherhood and the distinctive consciousness engendered by the material realities of life for black women. While our findings are consistent with hers, we would emphasize that this attitude exists, not only among African Americans, but among European Americans as well. The reasons for this resistance are rooted in shared values about the affective nature and noninstrumental significance of intimate relationships.

Conclusion: Context, Placebos, and Nocebos

It should now be clear that the major issue, the major concern, the major variable in all of these discussions about the ethics and social consequences of genetic disclosure is not whether information is disclosed, but the character of the social milieu into which that disclosure is disseminated. And the width and band of that social milieu is critical, from nation to culture to region to family unit. One family environment (or nation-state) may be safe and supportive for a child with Down syndrome, another quite hostile. It is not so much the disclosure that should occupy the focus of our analysis, but the context of that disclosure. As we have seen, under the highly commendable and politically safe banner of prospectively bringing greater health, molecular biologists "assume" that what they are doing will ultimately come down on the side of increasing public health (Hood 1992; Gilbert 1992).

However, the technology currently available in human molecular genetics is far more superior at diagnostics than at therapeutic interventions, and the prospects for the next decade all point to an increasing gap between diagnostics and therapeutics. To put it crisply, we are far better able to tell people what problems they are likely to encounter with genetic disorders than we are to intervene to reduce their health problems. In such a circumstance, "genetic disclosure" is primarily information provided about a condition that is strongly influenced by the genes, or a prospective future condition (even for potential offspring)—and in the circumstances described in this chapter, the issue of "nocebo effect" inevitably hovers over such disclosure.

The idea of placebo has only been in the lexicon of Western medicine for about fifty years. Before 1945, the term was not in general use, and could not be found in the title of an article for any medical journal (Weil 1988). However, it is now well established that if the subject believes that she or he has taken a medicine that might increase his or her health, under certain conditions that belief can alter conditions in the body:

Placebos can relieve severe postoperative pain, induce sleep or mental alertness, bring about dramatic remissions in both symptoms and objective signs of chronic disease, initiate the rejection of warts and other abnormal growths, and so forth. They can equally elicit all the undesired consequences of the treatment of drugs, including nausea, headaches, skin rashes, hives and more serious allergic reactions, damage to organs, and addictions. *In this case, they are sometimes called "nocebos" since their "effects" are noxious rather than pleasing* [italics mine] (Weil 1988, 209).

A genetic diagnosis of the kind described in this paper has all the elements needed for a "nocebo effect." Following Andrew Weil, one can certainly offer the quite plausible hypothesis that there will sometimes be a "nocebo effect" if the subject believes that there is "no hope" or no chance of a cure. As we have seen from findings for the research reported above, some family members "give up" hope for their children once they have been given a diagnosis of a genetic disorder, with an attendant spiral in a negative direction.[6]

One of the most promising areas for future research on the social consequences of genetic disclosure is in this arena: Is there a "nocebo effect" to the disclosure of a genetic predisposition, or carrier status, or disclosure of late-onset conditions? This is basically uncharted territory, and yet with the expanding diagnostic power of human molecular genetics, it is where we should focus more and more of our attention in the coming decades. We can begin to set up research programs to address this problem now, or we can trudge forward with the belief that someday, somehow, despite the increasing gap between what we can know and what we can heal, therapeutic intervention will make such research programs unnecessary.

Notes

1. The cost for an amniocentesis in India varies from 70 to 500 rupees (about $8 to $65), and the cost for an abortion is about the same (Rao 1988).

2. This is an unprecedented rate according to demographers who have been tracking such statistics around the world. Mobile units, buses, or even trucks can go into the rural areas, where nearly 80 percent of the Indian population lives ("India Fights Abortion of Female Fetuses," *New York Times*, August 27, 1994).

3. This refers to a development that was reported in the *New York Times*, November 14, 1993, entitled "China to Ban Sex Screening of Fetuses." Health Minister for

China, Chen Minzhang, announced the plan to enforce a new law that would not only prohibit screening of the fetus for sex determination, but also ban marriages for people "diagnosed with diseases that may totally or partially deprive the victim of the ability to live independently, that are highly possible to recur in generations to come and that are medically considered inappropriate for reproduction."

4. However, the Italians in the Bay Area of California have been displaying a level of "possessiveness" over the disease, and in one dramatic instance insisted that the term *Cooley's anemia* be preserved to distinguish the disease that people of Italian descent have and "not to confuse it" with the thalassemias of other populations.

5. This was a study carried out jointly under the direction of Diane Beeson and myself. The next section of this paper relies substantially on a segment of the final report of that work to the Department of Energy, which was the primary funding source.

6. The positive side of this remains the placebo; we have seen scores of families in which there has been a diagnosis of cystic fibrosis who rebounded with great hope at the prospects offered by placebos.

References

Draper, Elaine. 1991. *Risky Business: Genetic Testing and Exclusionary Practices in the Hazardous Workplace.* New York: Cambridge University Press.

Duster, Troy, and Diane Beeson. 1997. *Pathways and Barriers to Genetic Testing and Screening: Molecular Genetics Meets the "High-Risk Family."* Final Report, Office of Energy Research, Office of Health and Environmental Research of the U.S. Department of Energy, Washington, D.C.

Gilbert, Walter. 1992. A vision of the grail. In *The Code of Codes: Scientific and Social Issues in the Human Genome Project*, D. J. Kevles and L. Hood, eds., 96. Cambridge, Mass.: Harvard University Press.

Hill, Shirley A. 1994. Motherhood and the obfuscation of medical knowledge: The case of sickle cell disease. *Gender & Society* 8(1): 29–47.

Holtzman, Neil A. 1997. The second conference on genetics and primary care: The role of primary care providers and medical educators. In *Toward the 21st Century: Incorporating Genetics into Primary Health Care*, 7–11. Cold Spring Harbor, N.Y.: Cold Spring Harbor Press.

Holtzman, Neil A., and Michael S. Watson, eds. 1997. *Promoting Safe and Effective Genetic Testing in the United States: Final Report of the Task Force on Genetic Testing.* NIH DOE-Working Group on Ethical, Legal, and Social Implications of Human Genome Research. Bethesda, Md.: National Institutes of Health.

Hood, Leroy. 1992. Biology and medicine in the twenty-first century. In *The Code of*

Codes: Scientific and Social Issues in the Human Genome Project, D. J. Kevles and L. Hood, eds., 137–163. Cambridge, Mass.: Harvard University Press.

Kevles, D. J., and L. Hood. 1992. *The Code of Codes: Scientific and Social Issues in the Human Genome Project*. Cambridge, Mass.: Harvard University Press.

Lappé, M. 1988. Ethical issues in genetic screening for susceptibility to chronic lung disease. *J. Occup. Med.* 30: 493–501.

Nature. 1994. China's misconception of eugenics. *Nature* 367: 1.

Nelkin, Dorothy M., and Susan Lindee. 1995. *The DNA Mystique: The Gene as a Cultural Icon*. New York: Freeman.

New York Times. 1994. India fights abortion of female fetuses. (27 Aug.).

Rao, R. 1986. Move to stop sex-test abortion. *Nature* 32: 202.

Rao, R. 1988. Move to ban sex-determination. *Nature* 33: 467.

Weil, Andrew. 1988. *Health and Healing*. Boston: Houghton Mifflin.

9   The Fate of the Responsible Self in a Genetic Age

Ronald A. Carson, Ph.D.

Rapid growth in the volume of genetic information will soon outstrip medicine's therapeutic capabilities. Molecular genetics is booming. The hunt for genes for this disease and that condition continues to draw media attention. Patients are approaching doctors for tests they have heard about, often before their doctors know of their availability or purpose. What Evelyn Fox Keller calls "the discourse of gene action" is in rapid ascendance among biomedical scientists and the public alike (1995, 35). What are the legitimate uses of new genetic knowledge for modifying human behavior? Are there illicit uses? How would one decide? What are the implications of the new confidence that genes influence our behavior and shape our moral selves? What is the likely fate of the self in a genetic age?[1]

In premodern parlance, fate implied immutability and ruin; it was a sentence of the gods. Remnants of fatalistic thinking are reappearing with the discovery of genes associated with various diseases and conditions, especially those with behavioral components. It matters little that a sophisticated understanding of human existence must take into account the complex interaction of natural, cultural, and social factors.[2] Genetic determinism is predicated on the belief that what happens for genetic reasons is involuntary. It just happens. The Human Genome Project, on the other hand, is driven by the modern dream of mastering fate. Reductionist molecular science harbors a hopeful vision of a world in which the genetic bases of many diseases and their behavioral manifestations will be discovered and therapeutically prevented or treated.[3] It is a noble dream, though not unproblematic for our moral self-understanding. The tension between these two tendencies—our sense of our lives as fated, and the desire for mastery of what ails us—tugs at our understanding of ourselves as actors in the morality play of life.

Contra Automatic Utopianism

More than twenty-five years ago Hans Jonas recorded some prescient reflections on what he called "the new tasks of ethics" (Jonas 1973). Premodern ethics, Jonas observed, though not monomorphic, set out from some basic beliefs: that the human condition was given; that the range of human action for good or ill was therefore narrowly circumscribed; and that, in that light, the human good was "known in its generality" (Jonas 1973, 38) and largely uncontroversial. However, with the advent of modern science and our acquisition of novel technological powers, the nature of human action changed. "The qualitatively novel nature of certain of our actions has opened up a whole new dimension of ethical relevance for which there is no precedent in the standards and canons of traditional ethics" (Jonas 1973, 31).

In a world in which the circumstances of the human condition were believed to be largely impervious to human intervention, "the question was only how to relate to the stubborn fact" (Jonas 1973, 46). However, as we moderns acquired the knowledge and exercised the power to improve our lot, the human condition turned out to be more malleable than we had thought—a promising prospect and a problematic one in that decisions now had to be made without the comforting constraints of metaphysical and moral constancy. "The promised gift raises questions that had never to be asked before in terms of practical choice, and ... no principle of former ethics, which took the human constants for granted, is competent to deal with them" (Jonas 1973, 48). The new task of ethics in this situation is to counter the drift toward what Jonas calls "automatic utopianism" (Jonas 1973, 50)—doing something because it is doable and at the moment seems desirable, with little or no thought for its worthwhileness in the long run and in a larger scheme of things.

This metaphoric way of speaking is itself not unproblematic. We are having difficulty discerning responsible uses of new genetic information in part because a scheme of things larger than enclaves of likemindedness seems to elude us. Alasdair MacIntyre famously argued that what passes for moral pluralism in modern culture is actually mass confusion (1981). When one asks after the character of moral debates in our culture, what stands out is their interminability. Rival arguments, reaching mutually incompatible conclusions, bypass each other because they start from radically different premises. We possess no widely shared notion of how one goes about choosing among rival premises. MacIntyre claims that modern moral disagreements display three salient characteristics. First, arguments abound about moral merits and dangers (of, for example, attempting to alter violent behavior through genetic manipulation) and arrive at mutually incompatible conclusions. Each argument is logically valid on its own terms, but we have no widely agreed-upon method for weighing the rival claims of each. Second, these arguments purport to be impartial, that is, they claim to be authoritative by virtue of their appeal to rational principles rather than to subjective opinion. Third, what is imprecisely called pluralism in moral life and discourse masks a deep-seated conceptual confusion.

In a line of reasoning compatible with that of Jonas, MacIntyre observes that although our predecessors debated the great moral issues of their time and disagreed over, for example, whether the taking of human life was permissible, their assumptive worlds tended to be intact. We have inherited from them fragmented moral beliefs that are incoherent because they are detached from the intellectual and social contexts in which they were meaningful. This state of affairs inclines us to elevate an atomistic view of the self and negative liberty—the right to be left alone—above other values. One reasons thus: In a fragmented moral world, assuming I have the resources to carry out my wishes or to retain the services of an expert to execute my wishes, who is better qualified than I and those closest to me to decide what is best for me and mine, for example, in choosing the optimal optional characteristics of my unborn child? If the fragmented nature of our moral lives renders us powerless to make responsible decisions in accordance with some larger scheme of things, what alternative is there to leaving things up to individuals?

Such "libertarianism by default"[4] evokes calls for a reinstatement of the notion of taboo, the idea that some things are morally repugnant because they are inimical to human welfare. But by whose lights? "Repugnance," writes Leon Kass, "is the emotional expression of deep wisdom. . . . we intuit and feel, immediately and without argument, the violation of things that we rightfully hold dear" (Kass, 1997, 20).[5] Though they are effective among moral familiars, in the larger public arena, invocations of repugnance depend precisely on the shared sense of the limits of permissible action that we seem to lack. In a world where reproductive freedom is tantamount to parental autonomy, it makes eminently good sense to want to genetically select the characteristics of one's offspring. If, nevertheless, I recoil at this prospect, if my intuition is that sincere though the desire may be, genetically engineering one's child does not seem like a good idea, am I experiencing anything other than a "gut reaction"? If there are others who feel this way too, is our shared intuition perhaps simply different from the shared view of, say, the couples who would like a tall, blond, blue-eyed boy, or a deaf child, like themselves?

The valorizers of choice would answer in the affirmative. I am not so sure. Although moral intuitions are fallible, they need not be idiosyncratic. We do in fact have shared reactions to certain ideas and experiences. Intuitions are not irrelevant to moral inquiry. At a time when so much bioethical thinking is preoccupied with considerations of competing interests and conflicting values, moral inquiry might well be enriched by delving more deeply into why things seem intuitively good or bad, fitting or inappropriate, to people.[6] To say that we consider something desirable or repugnant is an expression of our way of viewing the world. Although it does not settle the matter, the way we feel about a morally perplexing matter is as good a place as any to begin to inquire into it. What will such an inquiry be like?

It will be a dialogue, because moral knowledge is relational and responsive. Acquiring moral knowledge requires attentiveness to others. We recognize where we stand and why only in the mirror of others' perceptions of us. We are only in a position to appreciate what others think and, if persuaded, to expand our vision or change our minds, when our sense of ourselves as responsible is at risk. Moreover, such a dialogue will be no mere mental exercise but will be "situated,"[7] which is to say, with Jonas, responsive to "the pressure of real habits of action" (Jonas 1973, 53). In our case these habits emanate from new genetic knowledge and the novel powers to use that knowledge in sometimes unpredictable and irreversible ways.

The Dialogical Self

Charles Taylor writes of the dialogical self that "we cannot understand human life merely in terms of individual subjects, who frame representations about and respond to others, because a great deal of human action happens only insofar as the agent understands and constitutes himself or herself as integrally part of a 'we.' Much of our understanding of self, society, and world is carried in practices that consist in dialogical action" (1994, 311).

The self is a concept so close to us as to be almost imperceptible. It is my "me," usually implying me at my truest, and that in two senses. In one sense, the self is thought to be free—not unfettered, but free to choose—and therefore accountable. Personal agency implies personal responsibility. In another sense, the self is believed to be integral—centered, however fragilely. The most persuasive evidence of this is that most of us, most of the time, go about our business with a sense of the general reliability of persons and things. Our confidence that the ordinary circumstances of our lives tomorrow are likely to be more or less continuous with the way they were today goes unquestioned. However, this confidence is not unshakable. It must be maintained against a background awareness of all that can go wrong in a risk-ridden culture such as ours. The proliferation of the popular notion that one may be characterologically predestined or genetically predisposed to behave in certain ways is likely to heighten that awareness and threaten the taken-for-grantedness of one's personal life.[8] What is the origin of this sense of the self as cohering in a livable way?

The moral ideal animating the modern idea of the self as a character type is that of being true to oneself and to others. The injunction, "to thine own self be true," expressed an aspiration to trustworthiness, the perception that one could be counted on to be constant in one's dealings with others. In a masterly account of the evolution of this ideal, Lionel Trilling has shown how sincerity became a defining characteristic of Western conceptions of culture and the self from the sixteenth century through the nineteenth century and how, with the dawning of modern self-consciousness, sincerity, up until then considered the absence of pretense—"a congruence between avowal and actual feeling"—was called into question by a new psychological awareness of the self's capacity to fool itself (Trilling, 1971, 7). Sincerity became suspect as an essential condition of virtue, but the desire to be true to oneself did not wane. This moral ideal henceforth assumed a new form, that of authenticity, "suggesting a more strenuous moral experience than 'sincerity' does, a more exigent conception of the self and of what being true to it consists in" (Trilling, 1971, 11).

With the rise of modernity, not only did the human condition seem newly malleable, as Jonas observed, but the idea of the self as given and discoverable was discredited. To be true to oneself now required more than "getting in touch" with oneself and maintaining self-alignment. It required moral work. One had to work at becoming one's "own original actual self" (Trilling, 1971, 10). Whereas the ideal of sincerity commended to the self a stance of compliance with the laws of nature and culture, the ideal of authenticity is adversarial, requiring what Trilling called "powers of indignant perception" with which to get to the root of received opinion to discern the inner workings of habitual ways of thinking. "There have always been selves. . . . Yet the self that makes itself manifest at the end of the eighteenth century is different in kind, and in effect, from any self that had ever before emerged. It is different in several notable respects, but there is one distinguishing characteristic which seems to me pre-eminently important: its intense and adverse imagination of the culture in which it has its being. [Culture] is the word by which we refer not only to a people's achieved work of intellect and imagination but also to its mere assumptions and unformulated valuations, to its habits, its manners, and its superstitions. The modern self is characterized by certain powers of indignant perception which, turned upon this unconscious portion of culture, have made it accessible to conscious thought" (Trilling 1979, i–ii).

The modern self is also a storied self. We become who we are by means of the conversations we carry on with each other about how things look to us and what life means to us from our various points of view. The self is our conception of ourselves as moral beings, a conception shaped and reshaped as we tell each other about, and recognize in each other, what matters most and least to us in life. We are particularly challenged when our well-rehearsed strategies for making ordinary decisions are interrupted, for example, by the discovery of information with fateful consequences about ourselves or our unborn children. "Fateful moments . . . stand in a particular relation to risk. They are moments at which the appeal of *fortuna* is strong, moments at which in more traditional settings, oracles might have been consulted or divine forces propitiated." Under conditions of modernity, we tend to consult experts, but even so, our sense of self-mastery is vulnerable because the decisions are ultimately ours to make (Giddens 1991, 113–114). Moreover, "risk, and risk calculation, edge aside *fortuna* in virtually all domains of human activity," with the consequence that "awareness of risk seeps into the actions of almost everyone" (Giddens 1991, 111–112). Such awareness, mitigated in premodern cultures by belief in tragedy or providence, awakens feelings of self-doubt and shame, both of which are forms of "anxiety about the adequacy of the narrative by means of which the individual sustains a coherent biography" (Giddens 1991, 65).[9] One feels personally insufficient, flawed, not up to the challenge of sustaining one's story line. This is not fear of something in particular but a free-floating anxiety prompted by the experience of what Nietzsche aptly termed "the weightlessness of all things"—an awareness of the risk of losing one's bearings in life.

The idea of the self is intelligible only by virtue of its place in a person's life story (was something someone did or said "in character," we ask).[10] I am born into stories that I did not invent; in some of them I will be a major character, in others play a minor role; in only one of them will I be the protagonist. My story will influence and limit your story and yours, mine. Our stories will have in common two characteristics. They will be open ended (and thus to an extent unpredictable) and lived toward certain futures and not others. It is in light of the knowledge of our individual and shared past and of our individual and collective vision of the future that we live our lives and then "edit" them.[11] We live narratively. We conceive our lives as having a beginning, middle, and (for the time being, temporary) end. There are highs and lows. We sometimes start over, but always within the context of what has gone before and what we expect to happen next, and after that. Subliminally aware of the tension between fate and mastery, we compare notes with each other in our mutual attempts to keep a coherent narrative going. Events and ideas that interrupt that identity-sustaining dialogue or threaten to weaken the powers of indignant perception that are its most valuable product should give us pause.

The New Task of Ethics

Hannah Arendt's probing analysis of the nature of human action provides insight into how moral identity can be maintained in the face of irreversibility and unpredictability. "The possible redemption from the predicament of irreversibility—of being unable to undo what one has done though one did not, and could not, have known what he was doing—is the faculty of forgiving. The remedy for unpredictability, for the chaotic uncertainty of the future, is contained in the faculty to make and keep promises. The two faculties belong together in so far as one of them, forgiving, serves to undo the deeds of the past" (Arendt 1959, 212–213).

Faced with the unpredictable ramifications of a therapeutic intervention based on behavioral genetics, our chief responsibility should be to refrain from making promises we are not sure we can keep. Only by cultivating our capacity to make and keep promises can we hope to maintain our sense of ourselves and each other as trustworthy and responsible. Because the future is uncertain, because the unforeseen and unforeseeable can destroy our promises, forgiveness too is necessary. Without it, our capacity to make new promises, to begin again, would be compromised. "Without being forgiven, released from the consequences of what we have done, our capacity to act would, as it were, be confined to one single deed from which we would never recover. . . . Without being bound to the fulfillment of promises, we would never be able to keep our identities" (Arendt 1959, 212–213).

These two faculties flourish or falter together. They could become reliable guides to us in our search for responsible uses of behavioral genetic knowledge, but only, it seems, if we can invent ways to keep promises into the unforeseeable future for which we are now responsible. Continuity between past and present was, of course, customarily sustained by tradition. We should revive this idea and ask ourselves how to expand our various traditions to encompass not only our ancestors and us but also our unborn descendants.[12]

Jonas concluded his ruminations on the new tasks of ethics by wondering "whether without restoring the category of the sacred, the category most thoroughly destroyed by the scientific enlightenment, we can have an ethics able to cope with the extreme powers which we possess today" (Jonas 1973, 52). It is a provocative question. Without an articulable notion of the sacred, how is one to know what counts as a violation?

Although vigilance in the face of temptations to hubris is always necessary, without a more widely shared sense of the sacred than our culture seems able to sustain, claims of sacrilege are likely to fall on deaf ears. However, if it makes sense to think of responsibility in narrative terms and as being possible only *in relation*, and assuming that our desire to be true to ourselves and each other has not slackened in this genetic age, it follows that we should encourage public narrative discourse to complement the exchange of stories by which we sustain our personal lives. We should talk with each other at every opportunity about what we think of new proposals to address a behavioral condition through genetic intervention, and probe each other's reasons for thinking the way we do. To avoid the shallowness of presentism, we should mine the stories we have inherited—religious traditions, civic traditions—for clues. We should, in short, cultivate moral reflection as a social capacity (Baier 1997, 41–63). By "we," I mean not only biomedical scientists and bioethicists, but also journalists and jurists, legislators, religious leaders, and policymakers, as well as members of an informed public—everyone, that is, who has a stake in the outcome of the dialogue about the fate of the responsible self in a genetic age.[13]

Ensuring this dialogue is the new task of ethics. The only alternative in sight is a tyranny of expertise.

Notes

1. Although I share concerns expressed by others about the likely implications of genetic accounts of human behavior for our understanding of individual responsibility, I will not consider here the question of how to hold free will and determinism

in creative tension (see Brock 1994, 18–33). Nor will I ponder the problem of "playing God." This phrase is often invoked by those for whom genetic research is tantamount to tampering with God's creation, an activity believed to be beyond the permissible bounds of human endeavor. However, these boundaries have long been fluid.

2. Susan M. Wolf (1995) provides a probing analysis of the concept of "geneticism."

3. Allan Brandt observed that "for any understanding of the relationship of culture and science, the problem of causation is critically important because it reflects directly on the question of responsibility for disease" (Brandt 1997, 85). Ruth Hubbard cautions against "the reductionist belief in genes as causes." "For more than a century people have been assured on scientific authority that the causes of our most serious personal and social problems reside within us. Now they are told that scientists soon will be able to cure all manner of ills—from sickle-cell anemia to manic depression and schizophrenia—by replacing 'bad genes' with 'good' ones. . . . Genes are only part of this story, and their roles are not sufficiently well understood to predict what will happen if one or another of them is changed, replaced, or even just moved from one position to another on the chromosomes" (Hubbard 1990, 82–83).

4. For a defense, see Engelhardt and Wildes (1994, 61–71). Also relevant is Robertson (1996).

5. See also Shattuck (1996). Instead of invoking the idea of taboo, Ted Peters develops a theological argument for the beneficent use of genetic science (1997).

6. Daniel Callahan (1994) makes a similar point in discussing what he calls conventional traditionalism. See also Gillett (1997, 239–245).

7. See Chapter 5 of Benhabib (1992, 158–177), especially the sections headed The Generalized versus the Concrete Other, and The 'Generalized' versus the 'Concrete' Other Reconsidered.

8. On modernity as a risk culture, see Giddens (1991 and 1990, especially Chapter 1).

9. In her memoir of living at risk for Huntington disease, Alice Wexler describes the "existential dilemma of living at risk" as involving "Magical, tormented thinking" (1995, xxii, 80).

10. "To imagine a person incapable of constitutive attachments . . . is not to conceive an ideally free and rational agent, but to imagine a person wholly without character, without moral depth. For to have character is to know that I move in a history I neither summon nor command, which carries consequences nonetheless for my choices and conduct" (Sandel 1984, 90).

11. "Unpredictability and teleology . . . coexist as part of our lives; like characters in a fictional narrative we do not know what will happen next, but none the less our lives have a certain form which projects itself toward our future" (MacIntyre 1981, 216).

12. I am grateful to Tom Cole for this insight.

13. Lest this seem an impractical suggestion, is should be noted that The Danish Council of Ethics has for more than a decade sponsored local "debate events," a cross between town meeting and focus group, on ethically controversial biomedical issues. These events have both contributed to the formation of policies responsive to public concern and provided a venue for the exercise of civic responsibility. For a related discussion of public science discourse as a means of constituting science as a public social activity, see Barns (1994).

References

Arendt, H. 1959. *The Human Condition*. Garden City, N.Y.: Doubleday Anchor Books.

Baier, A. C. 1997. *The Commons of the Mind*. Chicago: Open Court.

Barns, I. 1994. The Human Genome Project and the self. *Soundings* 77 (1–2) (Spring/Summer): 99–128.

Benhabib, S. 1992. *Situating the Self*. New York: Routledge.

Brandt, A. M. 1997. 'Just say no': Risk, behavior, and disease in twentieth century America. In *Scientific Authority and Twentieth Century America*, R. G. Walters, ed. Baltimore: Johns Hopkins University Press.

Brock, D. W. 1994. The Human Genome Project and human identity. In *Genes and Human Self-Knowledge*, R. F. Weir, S. W. Lawrence, and E. Fales, eds. Iowa City: University of Iowa Press.

Callahan, D. 1994. Manipulating human life: Is there no end to it? In *Medicine Unbound: The Human Body and the Limits of Medical Intervention*, R. H. Blank and A. L. Bonnicksen, eds., 118–131. New York: Columbia University Press.

Engelhardt, H. T., Jr., and K. W. Wildes. 1994. Postmodernity and limits on the human body. In *Medicine Unbound: The Human Body and the Limits of Medical Intervention*, R. H. Blank and A. L. Bonnicksen, eds. New York: Columbia University Press.

Giddens, A. 1990. *The Consequences of Modernity*. Stanford, Calif.: Stanford University Press.

Giddens, A. 1991. *Modernity and Self-Identify*. Stanford, Calif.: Stanford University Press.

Gillett, G. 1997. "We be of one blood, you and I": Commentary on Kopelman. In *Philosophy of Medicine and Bioethics*, R. A. Carson and C. R. Burns, eds. Boston: Kluwer Academic.

Hubbard, R. 1990. *The Politics of Women's Biology*. New Brunswick, N.J.: Rutgers University Press, 1990.

Jonas, H. 1973. Technology and responsibility: Reflections on the new tasks of ethics. *Soc. Res.* 40 (Spring): 31–54.

Kass, L. 1997. The wisdom of repugnance. *New Republic* 216(22): 17–26.

Keller, E. F. 1995. *Refiguring Life: Metaphors of Twentieth Century Biology.* New York: Columbia University Press.

MacIntyre, A. 1981. *After Virtue.* chaps. 1 and 2. Notre Dame, Ind.: University of Notre Dame Press.

Peters, T. 1997. *Playing God? Genetic Determinism and Human Freedom.* London: Routledge.

Robertson, J. A. 1996. Genetic selection of offspring characteristics. *Boston University Law Rev.* 73 (3) (June): 421–482.

Sandel, M. J. 1984. The procedural republic and the unencumbered self. *Political Theory* 12 (1) (Feb.): 81–96.

Shattuck, R. 1996. *Forbidden Knowledge: From Prometheus to Pornography.* New York: St. Martin's Press.

Taylor, C. 1994. The dialogical self. In *The Interpretive Turn,* D. Hiley, ed. Ithaca, N.Y.: Cornell University Press.

Trilling, L. 1971. *Sincerity and Authenticity.* Cambridge, Mass.: Harvard University Press.

Trilling, L. 1979. *The Opposing Self.* New York: Harcourt Brace Jovanovich (1955).

Wexler, A. 1995. *Mapping Fate.* Berkeley: University of California Press, 1995.

Wolf, S. M. 1995. Beyond "genetic determinism": Toward the broader harm of geneticism. *J. Law Med. Ethics* 23: 345–353.

Index

academic failure, 164–65

addiction, punishment for disease of, 122–24

adversary system of law, 102–4

affected individual and genetic disease disclosure, 179–81

affected pedigree member method of linkage analysis, 42

affected social group and ownership of genetic disease, 178–79

affecteds-only analysis, 49

aggression: consequences of finding genetic component of, 96–97; lead level and, 97, 160; MAOA deficiency and, 116–17, 118; as medical problem, 132; parental negativity and adolescent antisocial behavior, 27–28; popularity of genetic explanations of, 158–60; punishment of, 121–22, 126–27; violence prevention programs, 131–32

alcoholism: consequences of finding genetic component of, 95–96; as genetic defense, 126–27, 139; punishment for, 123–24; vulnerability to, vii–viii

allele-sharing methods, 41–42, 50–52, 68

allelic expansion, 92

allelic heterogeneity, 92

Alzheimer disease, 53

analysis of covariance, 26–28

anthropology, rejection of behavioral genetics by field of, 13

antisocial acts. See aggression; prediction and prevention of antisocial acts

anxiety, 52–53, 55

Arendt, Hannah, 195

Army Alpha Test, 90–91, 99–100

attachment theory, 23

attention deficit hyperactivity disorder (ADHD), 54–55

attitudes toward genetics, ix–x, 2–3. See also popular appeal of biological determinism

automatic utopianism, 190–92

Baker v. State Bar of California (1989), 126–27, 139

behavioral genetic model, 19–25

behavioral genetics: acceptance of, 12, 13, 14–16, 156; description of, 12

behavioral traits, correlation of genotype with, 93–98

Behavior Genetics Association, 12, 13, 14, 15, 156

Bell Curve, The (Herrnstein and Murray, 1994): controversy over, x, 61, 94, 95; genetic determinism and, 2; immigration and, 161–62; opposition to special education and affirmative action based on, 165; social trend of vindictiveness in, 127

Binet, Alfred, 90

biological determinism. See deterministic thinking

biological vulnerability, routes to, viii

biologists and genetic research, 3–5

biometric model-fitting analytic methods, 37–38

blame in families, 167–69, 182–85

blood pressure, 24

Born to Rebel (Sulloway, 1996), 7

Breakefield, Xandra, 116

Buck v. Bell (1927), 98–99

C. (Caenorhabditis) elegans: limitations in use of, 73–76; as model organism, 71–73

Caldwell v. State (1987), 125–26, 140

Calvinist Protestants, 8–9

cancer, viewed as genetic disease, 167

Printed in the United States
4821

Made in the USA
Lexington, KY
26 July 2011